Schizophrenia and Related Disorders

Schizophrenia and Related Disorders

Edited by

Michael J. Marcsisin, MD

Assistant Professor
Department of Psychiatry
University of Pittsburgh School of Medicine

Jessica M. Gannon, MD

Assistant Professor
Department of Psychiatry
University of Pittsburgh School of Medicine

Jason B. Rosenstock, MD

Associate Professor
Department of Psychiatry
University of Pittsburgh School of Medicine
Director, Medical Student Education
Western Psychiatric Institute and Clinic

OXFORD
UNIVERSITY PRESS

OXFORD
UNIVERSITY PRESS

Oxford University Press is a department of the University of Oxford. It furthers
the University's objective of excellence in research, scholarship, and education
by publishing worldwide. Oxford is a registered trade mark of Oxford University
Press in the UK and certain other countries.

Published in the United States of America by Oxford University Press
198 Madison Avenue, New York, NY 10016, United States of America.

Library of Congress Cataloging-in-Publication Data
Names: Marcsisin, Michael J., editor. | Gannon, Jessica M., editor. |
    Rosenstock, Jason, editor.
Title: Schizophrenia and related disorders / edited by Michael J. Marcsisin,
    Jessica M. Gannon, Jason B. Rosenstock.
Other titles: Pittsburgh pocket psychiatry series.
Description: Oxford ; New York : Oxford University Press, [2016] | Series:
    Pittsburgh pocket psychiatry series | Includes bibliographical references.
Identifiers: LCCN 2016009493 (print) | LCCN 2016010135 (ebook) |
    ISBN 9780199331505 (pbk. : alk. paper) | ISBN 9780199331512 (U-pdf) |
    ISBN 9780199331529 (Epub)
Subjects: | MESH: Schizophrenia
Classification: LCC RC514 (print) | LCC RC514 (ebook) | NLM WM 203 |
    DDC 616.89/8—dc23
LC record available at http://lccn.loc.gov/2016009493

9 8 7 6 5 4 3 2 1

Printed by Sheridan Books, Inc., United States of America

Series Introduction

We stand on the threshold of a new golden age of clinical and behavioral neuroscience with psychiatry at its fore. With the Pittsburgh Pocket Psychiatry series, we intend to encompass the breadth and depth of our current understanding of human behavior in health and disease. Using the structure of resident didactic teaching, we will be able to ensure that each subject area relevant to practicing psychiatrists is detailed and described. New innovations in diagnosis and treatment will be reviewed and discussed in the context of existing knowledge, and each book in the series will propose new directions for scientific inquiry and discovery. The aim of the series as a whole is to integrate findings from all areas of medicine and neuroscience previously segregated as "mind" or "body," "psychological" or "biological." Thus, each book from the Pittsburgh Pocket Psychiatry series will stand alone as a standard text for anyone wishing to learn about a specific subject area. The series will be the most coherent and flexible learning resource available.

David Kupfer, MD
Michael Travis, MD
Michelle Horner, DO

Contents

Contributors

Jaspreet S. Brar, MD, PhD
Department of Psychiatry
University of Pittsburgh
School of Medicine
Western Psychiatric Institute
and Clinic
Pittsburgh, Pennsylvania

Shaun M. Eack, PhD
University of Pittsburgh
School of Social Work
Pittsburgh, Pennsylvania

Justin C. Ellison, PharmD, BCPP
Department of Pharmacy
University of Pittsburgh
School of Pharmacy
Western Psychiatric Institute
and Clinic
Pittsburgh, Pennsylvania

Jessica M. Gannon, MD
Department of Psychiatry
University of Pittsburgh
School of Medicine
Western Psychiatric Institute
and Clinic
Pittsburgh, Pennsylvania

Gil D. Hoftman, MD, PhD
Department of Psychiatry
University of Pittsburgh School
of Medicine
Western Psychiatric Institute
and Clinic
Pittsburgh, Pennsylvania

Michael J. Marcsisin, MD
Department of Psychiatry
University of Pittsburgh School
of Medicine
Western Psychiatric Institute
and Clinic
Pittsburgh, Pennsylvania

Konasale M. Prasad, MD
Department of Psychiatry
University of Pittsburgh School
of Medicine
Western Psychiatric Institute
and Clinic
Pittsburgh, Pennsylvania

Jason B. Rosenstock, MD
Department of Psychiatry
University of Pittsburgh School
of Medicine
Western Psychiatric Institute
and Clinic
Pittsburgh, Pennsylvania

Dean F. Salisbury, PhD
Department of Psychiatry
University of Pittsburgh School
of Medicine
Western Psychiatric Institute
and Clinic
Pittsburgh, Pennsylvania

History and Phenomenology of Schizophrenia and Related Psychoses

Michael J. Marcsisin and Jessica M. Gannon

Introduction and Overall Approach

Maybe each human being lives in a unique world, a private world different from those inhabited and experienced by all other humans. . . . If reality differs from person to person, can we speak of reality singular, or shouldn't we really be talking about plural realities? And if there are plural realities, are some more true (more real) than others? What about the world of a schizophrenic? Maybe it's as real as our world. Maybe we cannot say that we are in touch with reality and he is not, but should instead say, His reality is so different from ours that he can't explain his to us, and we can't explain ours to him. The problem, then, is that if subjective worlds are experienced too differently, there occurs a breakdown in communication . . . and there is the real illness.

—Philip K. Dick

History is a collection of experiences, a defining narrative that lends itself to a better understanding of our present. Knowing the history of an illness allows practitioners to better appreciate its manifestations, its diagnostic challenges, and most importantly, its impact on the people whose lives have been touched by its presence. Phenomenology is rooted in history. It is a detailed, comprehensive collection of signs and symptoms observed and reported in psychiatric conditions. Phenomenology can also be defined as the study of patients' subjective experiences of a disorder, which in and of itself is rooted in history and culture. As mental health providers, we seek to learn about the phenomenology and history of mental illness, as it is essential for us to recognize the signs and symptoms of a disorder and respect that they represent unique experiences lived by our patients and are heavily affected by historical and cultural context. So often the inner world and behaviors of someone with a schizophrenia spectrum illness can seem remote and inaccessible to us and challenge our empathy. To know the phenomenology and appreciate the history of schizophrenia and related psychoses is to possess a framework of understanding, a way to grasp the unique struggles of patients, so as to facilitate truly patient-centered care.

A History of Schizophrenia Spectrum Disorders

Schizophrenia is a broad clinical syndrome defined by reported subjective experiences, loss of functioning, and a variable course. It has a complex etiology and is clearly influenced by both genetic and environmental factors. The concept of schizophrenia as a medical illness is a product of the late nineteenth and early twentieth centuries, but the behaviors and disorders in functioning characteristic of schizophrenia spectrum disorders have existed since ancient times. While psychosis, in some form, has probably been present since ancient times, there is much controversy surrounding the origins of schizophrenia itself, so this chapter will focus on the history of this psychotic disorder in particular.

Accounts of "madness" or insanity can be found as far back as ancient Egypt and probably represent the manifestations of a number of conditions, some of which may meet criteria for modern mental disorders. Retrospective diagnosis is difficult, however, and is limited by missing data, the imposition of our current understanding of disease onto past conceptualizations, and varying diagnostic criteria, as well as by stigma and other cultural biases (Fraguas & Breathnach, 2009). Some scholars believe that schizophrenia is an ancient illness, and evidence for this hypothesis is outlined in this chapter. Others maintain that the disorder did not begin to manifest until the seventeenth or eighteenth centuries (Jeste et al., 1985). Some such theorists have argued that schizophrenia may have a modern-age viral vector, as convincing accounts of the illness did not exist before the pre-industrial, urbanization age when large groups of people began living in closer quarters. These critics also point to the apparently rising number of cases of schizophrenia in the modern era while simultaneously emphasizing the relatively low fertility rate of people with this disorder (Hare, 1988). If schizophrenia was a longstanding genetic disorder, why would its prevalence seemingly have increased during industrialization? Others postulate that schizophrenia-like illness has existed for centuries, but that our understanding of this illness as "schizophrenia" is a product of our own culture and time.

Ancient descriptions of madness can be read in religious texts like the Bible and the Hindu Vedas, as well as in early medical texts, including the Egyptian *Ebers Papyrus* and the Chinese *The Yellow Emperor's Classic of Internal Medicine*. Greek and Roman literature also references madness. In these early writings, the descriptions of madness widely vary and are often attributed to spiritual disturbances: including, but not limited to, demonic possession. The Greeks and Romans sometimes allowed for more biological explanations of madness, generally relating to the Greek theory of the imbalance of "humors," and they unambiguously recognized symptoms of hallucinations and delusions. However, reviewers of Greek and Roman depictions of madness have not found definitive evidence of schizophrenia, as they have not been able to convincingly meet retrospective diagnostic criteria for the illness.

In the Middle Ages, schizophrenia may have been treated by medieval Islamic physicians, most notably Ibn Sina, who described madness as a break from reality accompanied by behavioral disturbances, agitation, alterations in sleep, and difficulty with communication. He, as well as many of his contemporaries, theorized that madness was caused by a disturbance in the brain, and in many cases was hereditary. Ibn Sina further recognized mania as a separate illness. Islamic hospitals that cared for the seriously mentally ill began to spring up as early as the ninth century, and restraints were often used, seemingly to prevent patients from harming themselves or others. As such, it may have been that people who could not care for themselves, and who were potentially violent, were the most likely to be classified as mad. On the other hand, in both the Middle East and Europe, individuals who had probable hallucinations and delusions, but were not violent, may have been revered as mystics, saints, or other respected religious figures.

Europeans of the Middle Ages and the Enlightenment period were familiar with madness, as evidenced by literary classics like Shakespeare's *King Lear* and Cervantes's *Don Quixote*. Descriptions of historical figures like the eighteenth-century sculptor Franz Xaver Messerschmidt, who seemed to suffer from hallucinations of demons and delusions of persecution, and Opicinus de Canistris, the fourteenth-century Italian scribe who spent decades in solitude working on strange maps, have been well explored in the literature as possible case reports of schizophrenia. The first asylums for individuals with madness or insanity began opening in Europe in the 1200s. Monasteries often cared for the mentally ill prior to this, as did some more general hospitals, like Paris's seventh-century Hôtel-Dieu, which later became an asylum. London's Priory of Saint Mary of Bethlehem, later known as the Bethlem Royal Hospital, and colloquially as

"Bedlam," opened in 1285, and a string of asylums opened across Spain in the 1400s. By the 1700s, private and public hospitals for the mentally ill had spread across the European nations and their colonies, and the public gradually became aware of, and appalled by, the abuse and neglect of the patients that too often came with these institutions. This public sentiment helped support the early to mid–nineteenth-century reforms of William Tuke in England and Philippe Pinel and Jean-Baptiste Pussin in France, who famously freed their patients from their chains, ushering in the heyday of "moral treatment." Pinel was also an early champion of formal diagnoses of insanity, and he was one of the first physicians to attempt to classify patients' illnesses, not only by symptoms, but by course.

Did the patients in these early asylums have schizophrenia? The answer is uncertain. Pinel wrote of adolescent patients with "dementia," some of whom had features of the later "dementia praecox," the diagnosis most closely associated with the modern diagnosis of schizophrenia. In England, Pinel's contemporary George Mann Burrows wrote of an adolescent-onset disorder leading to "chronic demency," describing a thought disorder with difficulties in "associating and comparing ideas" and "arranging thoughts." However, he linked this condition closely with affective disturbance. The prominent director of the Bethlem, John Haslan, similarly wrote of an adolescent-onset disorder leading to cognitive disintegration, avolition, and apathy, but also with mood lability with intermittent aggression. Haslan is known for his sometimes controversial work, including with the famed patient James Tilly Matthews, starting in 1809, who had chronic persecutory delusions and is considered by many to have the first convincingly documented case of schizophrenia.

In the 1840s, Wilhelm Griesinger wrote of types of dementia and chronic mania that appear to overlap with modern schizophrenia diagnoses. At the same time, Griesinger, like his contemporary Ernst Zeller, and more radically, Heinrich Neumann, embraced the concept of a "unitary psychosis," espousing the concept that all forms of insanity were caused by the same endogenous disorder.

The end of the nineteenth century, however, heralded the beginning of a new era in the diagnosis and treatment of mental illness. German physicians like Karl Ludwig Kahlbaum and his disciple, Ewald Hecker, laid the groundwork for the modern conceptualization of mental illness, breaking away from the theory of unitary psychosis. Symptom patterns and features like age of onset, family history, course, and age of outcome became increasingly important. It was in this environment that Emil Kraepelin began his study of patients with mental illness.

Emil Kraepelin is often considered the father of biological psychiatry and the modern nosological approach to defining and categorizing individual psychiatric illnesses. Working and writing in the late nineteenth century, Kraepelin was the first person to identify and classify what we have come to know as "schizophrenia" as an illness distinct from other major psychiatric disorders. Using comprehensive clinical observations, Kraepelin proposed that "dementia praecox" (dementia of the young) was a chronic illness starting in adolescence and early adulthood that led to an inevitable deterioration in behavior and functioning. Kraepelin distinguished dementia praecox with its frequently chronic, downward course, from the "affective psychoses"—unipolar and bipolar depression—which he believed were more variable in their clinical course and better in their prognosis and outcome. In rejecting the concept of a unitary psychosis, Kraepelin did not presume to identify the etiological factors or create diagnostic criteria for these disorders, but he did believe his work in clinical categorization would lead to, and be validated by, advances in the scientific understanding of these "diseases of the brain."

Following Kraepelin, Eugen Bleuler was a Swiss psychiatrist who recognized the significance of dementia praecox as a physical illness but believed that the disorder was more heterogeneous than Kraepelin allowed. In 1908, Bleuler coined the term *schizophrenia* ("split mind") to replace dementia praecox. In so doing, he revised and expanded the concept of schizophrenia. For Kraepelin, the key feature of dementia praecox was its "terminal state" of deterioration—anyone having dementia praecox had a poor outcome with no chance of recovery. Bleuler, on the other hand, saw schizophrenia as a "group of diseases" with key and common "basic" symptoms and a more variable course and prognosis. He identified these key "basic" symptoms as disordered thought and speech (loosening of associations), volitional indeterminacy (ambivalence), affective incongruence, and withdrawal from reality (autism). These key symptoms have come to be known as "Bleuler's Four A's" and are what made schizophrenia (for Bleuler) distinct from other psychiatric illnesses. Bleuler also identified accessory or supplementary symptoms—delusions and hallucinations—which are common to his concept of schizophrenia but not its defining feature. These accessory symptoms are the "positive symptoms" of the current diagnostic criteria for schizophrenia.

Kurt Schneider further revised and elaborated upon the concept of schizophrenia by identifying what have come to be known as "Schneiderian First-Rank symptoms." Schneider believed certain symptoms were characteristic of schizophrenia and were therefore particularly significant in clinical diagnosis. These symptoms include auditory hallucinations in which the individual hears voices speaking to each other or commenting on the actions of the individual; delusions of being controlled by an external force; delusions that the individual's thoughts are being inserted or withdrawn by others or that the individual is broadcasting his thoughts to others; and delusional perceptions from which the individual would draw a bizarre conclusion from otherwise normal sensory perceptions. These First-Rank symptoms greatly contributed to the modern conceptualization of schizophrenia. In *The Diagnostic and Statistical Manual of Mental Disorders*' third and fourth editions (DSM-III and DSM-IV), the presence of any of these symptoms was considered sufficient to diagnose schizophrenia. In contrast, in DSM-5, Schneiderian First-Rank symptoms are no longer emphasized or considered sufficient to make a diagnosis of schizophrenia, as recent studies have called into question the diagnostic specificity of these symptoms to the disorder.

In 1950, French chemist Paul Charpentier, while attempting to develop improved antihistamines, synthesized the first effective medical treatment for psychotic illnesses: chlorpromazine (for more information on chlorpromazine and other somatic treatments, see Chapter 6 of this text). Used initially to enhance anesthesia, chlorpromazine was found to have a calming effect on surgical patients. Pierre Deniker and Jean Delay, psychiatrists at the Hôpital Sainte-Anne in Paris, heard of chlorpromazine's calming effects and ordered samples of the medication to give to 38 psychotic and agitated patients. The resulting clinical trial, published in 1952, showed dramatic improvements in the behaviors and cognition of the trial patients and began a revolution in the treatment of schizophrenia and psychotic illnesses. For the first time, physicians had an effective medical treatment for schizophrenia; researchers recognized that it was possible to develop drugs to treat psychiatric illness; and patients with psychosis and their families had some hope that their symptoms could be alleviated and that they would not be confined indefinitely. In 1954, chlorpromazine was licensed for use in the United States as Thorazine. Over the next 30 years, the use of Thorazine and similar antipsychotic medications helped facilitate the deinstitutionalization of psychiatric patients, with the number of patients confined to state and county hospitals in the United States dropping from approximately 560,000 in 1955 to under 30,000 in the early 2000s.

During the 1960s and 1970s, controversies arose over the concept and diagnostic validity of "schizophrenia." In a movement that has come to be known as "Anti-Psychiatry," psychiatrists and social scientists, including Thomas Szasz, R. D. Laing, Erving Goffman, and Michel Foucault, challenged the idea of mental illness itself, arguing that schizophrenia in particular was an artificial construct that lacked a scientific basis and was used to repress or marginalize society's poor and nonconformists. Academic psychiatrists and researchers acknowledged the lack of indisputable scientific evidence at that time for schizophrenia. They further expressed concern that the diagnostic criteria for schizophrenia were problematically unclear, such that schizophrenia was not consistently or reliably diagnosed. This concern was highlighted by David Rosenhan's study in 1972, *On Being Sane in Insane Places*, which found the diagnostic criteria used in the United States were often subjective and unreliable and led to more diagnoses of "Schizophrenia" in the United States than elsewhere.

As the Anti-Psychiatry movement was taking shape, a group of academic psychiatrists at Washington University in St. Louis, Missouri, was working on methods to improve the validity and reliability of psychiatric diagnoses. This group, which included Eli Robins, Samuel Guze, John Feighner, and George Winokur, argued that researchers could not hope to make scientific advances in the pathophysiology and treatment of psychiatric illness until psychiatrists and researchers reached a consensus on what constituted psychiatric illness and could reliably diagnose psychiatric disorders. Their work led to the 1972 publication in the *Archives of General Psychiatry,* "Diagnostic Criteria for Use in Psychiatric Research"—now commonly known as the "Feighner Criteria" for psychiatric diagnoses.

The Feighner Criteria are significant in the history of psychiatry in general, and of schizophrenia in particular, because they became the basis for DSM-III, -IV, and -5. Until the publication of the Feighner Criteria, psychiatric diagnosis was inconsistent and based largely on general and vague descriptions of psychiatric illness. The DSM-II entry on schizophrenia, for example, describes the illness in general terms, lists and describes 10+ subtypes, but offers little guidance on how to diagnose the illness:

> This large category includes a group of disorders manifested by characteristic disturbances of thinking, mood, and behavior. Disturbances in thinking are marked by alterations of concept formation which may lead to misinterpretation of reality and sometimes to delusions and hallucinations, which frequently appear psychologically self-protective. Corollary mood changes include ambivalent, constricted, and inappropriate emotional responsiveness and loss of empathy with others. Behavior may be withdrawn, regressive, and bizarre. The schizophrenias, in which the mental status is attributable primarily to a thought disorder, are to be distinguished from the Major affective illnesses (q.v.) which are dominated by a mood disorder. (1968, p. 33)

In contrast, the Feighner Criteria introduced the systematic use of operationalized diagnostic criteria for psychiatric illness, emphasized the importance of illness course and outcome, and reintroduced to psychiatry the idea that diagnostic criteria for psychiatric illnesses must be grounded in empirical evidence. These concepts had been recognized among psychiatrists like Kraepelin and Bleuler in the nineteenth and early twentieth centuries, but they had largely been eclipsed in the United States in the mid-twentieth century by the rise and dominance of Freudian psychoanalytical psychiatry.

Similar to Kraepelin's concept of dementia praecox, the Feighner Criteria specify that schizophrenia is a chronic illness, without prominent mood symptoms, which leads to notable declines in functioning. Symptoms are evident for at least six months and include either delusions or hallucinations, or disorganized thought and communication. The illness starts before the age of 40 and is not influenced during the first year of onset by substance or alcohol abuse. The diagnostic criteria for schizophrenia under the Feighner Criteria are thus clearly specified, and individuals cannot be diagnosed with schizophrenia unless they meet a combination of these operational criteria.

The Feighner Criteria became the most cited paper in psychiatry in the 1970s and helped spur a revolution in the way mental illnesses are conceptualized and psychiatry is practiced. The Criteria were revised and expanded by Robert Spitzer and Eli Robins in their 1978 paper "Research Diagnostic Criteria: Rationale and Reliability" (or, as it has come to be known, "the Research Diagnostic Criteria"—RDC). The RDC made Schneiderian First-Rank symptoms prominent in the diagnosis of schizophrenia; it also separated the concept and diagnosis of schizoaffective disorder from schizophrenia. Together, the Feighner Criteria and the RDC emphasized what has been termed a "neo-Kraepelinian" approach to psychiatry, in which physicians follow a largely biomedical and longitudinal approach to observing, diagnosing, and treating the symptoms, signs, and course of mental illnesses.

In 1974, the American Psychiatric Association tacitly acknowledged the issues surrounding psychiatric diagnosis by convening a task force to revise and update DSM-II. Under the leadership of Robert Spitzer, the DSM-III task force was asked to create a new manual that would make psychiatric diagnoses explicit, reliable, and valid. Spitzer sought to accomplish this goal by building upon the Feighner Criteria and the RDC; it can be argued that the resulting DSM-III (and subsequent revisions in DSM-IV and -5) would not have been possible without the publication of the Feighner Criteria and the RDC.

DSM-III incorporates explicit operational criteria for all diagnoses and emphasizes the importance of evaluating the signs and symptoms of psychiatric illnesses longitudinally. Schizophrenia in DSM-III can be diagnosed when an individual meets criteria from three separate areas—characteristic symptoms, impairment, and chronicity—and does not have symptoms of the "full depressive or manic syndrome" prior to the onset of psychosis or an "Organic Mental Disorder." Characteristic symptoms relied heavily on Schneiderian First-Rank symptoms and were grouped into "characteristic delusions" (delusions of being controlled, thought broadcasting, thought insertion, thought withdrawal, bizarre delusions, somatic/grandiose/religious/nihilistic delusions, and any delusion accompanied by hallucinations), "characteristic hallucinations" (a single voice that provides a running commentary on an individual's behaviors/thoughts, or multiple voices that converse with each other, and hallucinations that have "no relation to depression or elation"), and "other characteristic symptoms" (incoherence, derailment, marked illogicality, poverty of content of speech). DSM-III specified that an individual could be diagnosed with schizophrenia if he displayed at least one of these characteristic symptoms, had significant impairments in at least two areas of "routine daily functioning," and had been symptomatic continuously for at least six months.

Subsequent editions of the DSM (III-R, IV, IV-TR, 5) have revised and simplified the criteria for schizophrenia, but the overall framework and approach established in DSM-III to evaluating and diagnosing individuals with schizophrenia remain essentially unchanged.

Phenomenology of Schizophrenia Spectrum Disorders

Schizophrenia

Schizophrenia is a complex disorder with myriad symptoms. Diagnosing schizophrenia can be relatively simple, as signs and symptoms are often readily identified that, in total, meet DSM criteria for the disorder. Diagnosis is a fundamental part of patient assessment, but in schizophrenia, a more comprehensive evaluation for signs and symptoms than what is needed for diagnosis should be completed. Identifying all symptoms that are potentially impairing for the patient, truly understanding the phenomenology of the illness, is key to providing patient-centered, informed treatment planning, especially as different symptoms are often targeted by different treatment modalities.

Symptoms of schizophrenia are often best understood by providers through the use of one of several classification systems, in which signs and symptoms of the disorder are grouped into clusters or domains of seemingly related signs and symptoms (Table 1.1). One major conceptualization organizes symptoms into positive, negative, and cognitive symptom clusters. Kaplan and Saddock textbooks classically present schizophrenia as a collection of positive symptoms, negative symptoms, and

Table 1.1 Example of Symptom Clustering

Positive Symptoms	"Extra" perceptions, thoughts, and behaviors not present in the absence of psychosis. Include hallucinations, delusions, bizarre or disorganized speech and behaviors, and agitation.
Negative Symptoms	A lack of normal thoughts, behaviors, and feelings. Includes anhedonia, avolition/passivity, asociality or social withdrawal, affective blunting (or flattening), alogia.
Cognitive Symptoms	Difficulties with attention, deficits in memory, abnormalities in executive functions, disorders of verbal fluency, and social cognitive deficits.

disorganization symptoms. The DSM-5 symptom domains for schizophrenia spectrum and other psychotic disorders are delusions, hallucinations, disorganized thinking (manifesting clinically as disorganized speech), grossly disorganized or abnormal motor behavior (including catatonia), and negative symptoms. The first three domains are considered "core positive symptoms;" a patient must have one these symptoms to ultimately meet criteria for a diagnosis of schizophrenia. The DSM also recognizes cognitive symptoms and affective symptoms, including depression, anxious mood, and even mania, as important aspects of the illness, though not essential to the diagnosis. Regardless of symptom classification, caution in organizing symptoms into clusters is fundamental, as symptom clusters can overlap and may not be inordinately useful in understanding the neurobiological or neuropsychological underpinnings of the disorder.

For ease of use for the active student practitioner, we will explore the phenomenology of schizophrenia by examining the DSM-5 symptom domains.

Delusions and Hallucinations

Delusions and hallucinations are the most widely recognized as "psychotic" symptoms. These symptoms, and the associated distress experienced by patients and their natural supports (family, friends, etc.), most often bring people with schizophrenia to the attention of medical providers. Importantly, these are also the symptoms that respond best to available pharmacological therapies. Hallucinations and delusions, in addition to grossly disorganized thoughts, speech, and behaviors, make up the bulk of DSM-5 Criterion A for a diagnosis of schizophrenia.

Hallucinations

Hallucinations are perceptual disturbances occurring in the absence of external stimuli and can be experienced as auditory, visual, gustatory, and/or tactile. Auditory hallucinations occur in up to 75% of people with schizophrenia. They can present at varying frequencies and levels of intensity and volume. These hallucinations are classically perceived by the patient as "voices," which can sound much like normal human voices, or can sound unnatural or even alien. Voices may be perceived as familiar, like those belonging to loved ones, peers, or persons of prominence or celebrity. They can also seem unfamiliar and be attributed to spiritual entities, extraterrestrials, or other imaginary characters. The voices may speak in whole sentences, parts of sentences, or utter a word or two. Schneiderian First-Rank symptoms, including voices that provide a commentary on a person's actions or refer to the sufferer in third person, are commonly experienced by those with schizophrenia but are not pathognomonic for the illness as once thought. Patients can experience auditory hallucinations other than voices, including hearing animal sounds or mechanical noises. In schizophrenia spectrum disorders, auditory hallucinations can be perceived as coming from inside or outside of the body, although many traditionally held that auditory hallucinations associated with schizophrenia were more likely to be perceived by sufferers as coming from an external location. The phenomenological features of any one patient's auditory hallucinations are subject to change throughout the often-varying course of their illness. It is worth noting that some people with schizophrenia only hear voices during periods of overall symptom exacerbation, while others experience auditory hallucinations more chronically.

Auditory hallucinations are perceived by patients to have negative, positive, or more neutral qualities, often depending on the tone or volume of the sounds heard or the content of a verbal message. If these qualities of the auditory hallucination are congruent with mood or thought content—i.e., voices are disparaging when the patient is upset with herself and thinking negatively—they can be called "ego syntonic." If there is dissonance between the patient's mood or thought content and the auditory hallucinations, like if the hallucinations are perceived as threatening but the patient feels euphoric, the auditory hallucinations would be considered "ego dystonic."

Auditory hallucinations can seem quite meaningful, or salient, to the patient. They can cause thus high levels of distress and deeply affect a person's ability to function. Auditory hallucinations can be very distracting to the patient trying to complete even the most basic of tasks, like cooking a meal or doing laundry. Patients sometimes feel that they should talk back to the voices or otherwise interact with them, causing them to mumble to themselves or yell out. Many patients suffering from intense auditory hallucinations will sometimes appear internally preoccupied, as they are focused on the auditory hallucinations to the exclusion of attaining to other stimuli. It may not be clear to the patient exactly why the voices they hear provoke such a strong emotional response and otherwise seem so important to them, leaving the patient searching for an explanation. It is thus common for auditory hallucinations to be incorporated into, or even drive, delusions. Over the course of the illness, many individuals with chronic auditory hallucinations gain the ability to ignore or otherwise successfully cope with many of their auditory hallucinations. Likewise, some individuals' hallucinations seem to become more pleasant and companionable over time, even guiding the patient, like an audible conscience or moral compass (Sadock et al., 2009). Many patients, however, continue to find the hallucinations bothersome and significantly impairing.

Command auditory hallucinations are experienced by patients as commanding them to perform actions. These types of hallucinations are not uncommon in schizophrenia and were experienced by 22% of patients in one study (Harkavy-Friedman et al., 2003). The commands are sometimes to perform actions that are unacceptable. Screening for these types of auditory hallucinations has long been considered to be important, since commands can, for instance, order the sufferer to harm themselves or others. There is some evidence that people with command auditory hallucinations to harm others are more likely to be violent (McNiel et al., 2000). Other studies show that patients with command auditory hallucinations to harm themselves are also more likely to do so (Harkavy-Freidman et al., 2003). There are other studies, though, that do not show any positive associations of command auditory hallucinations with violence toward self or others (Monahan et al., 2000). Understanding why some individuals with command auditory hallucinations seem more prone or compelled to act on them than others is an ongoing area of study.

Case Example

Vanessa is a 19-year-old Hispanic female diagnosed with schizophrenia. She presents to your psychiatric emergency room in some distress, intermittently sobbing. Based on a history you gather from her mother, who brought her in today, the patient has been complaining of hearing a multitude of voices, throughout the day, every day, for the last several weeks. This has affected her ability to sleep and to care for herself, with the patient's mother noting that the patient sits at home much of the time, mumbling to herself and otherwise seeming to interact with the voices. The patient has been having similar experiences with voices for the past year, but she notes that, lately, things are "much, much worse." She admits that has not been leaving the house or attending to her hygiene. Per her mother's report, the patient has told her that some of the voices scream profanities at her, and the patient appears alternately sad and frightened when she experiences this. The patient has also told her mother that she hears the voice of her deceased grandmother, who will say nice, comforting things. The patient's mother insisted she be urgently evaluated today as the patient told her just this morning that she is hearing a voice telling her to jump out into traffic, and that the cars won't harm her if she follows though. During the interview, the patient appears internally preoccupied, listening intently to something that you cannot hear and weeping, making it difficult to attend to you or her mother, complicating your examination.

Visual hallucinations are the second most common type of hallucinations experienced by those with schizophrenia spectrum disorders. About a third of patients with schizophrenia have visual hallucinations sometime during their illness (Sadock, 2009), and visual hallucinations may predict, or be indicative of, a more severe illness course (Teeple, Caplan, & Stern, 2009). Much care should be afforded in differential diagnostic considerations of those with visual hallucinations, as these hallucinations are commonly experienced by patients with substance intoxication or withdrawal or specific medical conditions (e.g., seizure disorder, migraines, brain tumors, etc.). Delirium is a medical condition that very commonly presents with visual hallucinations, and this presentation is likely to be familiar to those with medical training. As people with schizophrenia may develop delirium with medical illnesses, it is useful to appreciate the phenomenological differences between the visual hallucinations of these two conditions. Classically, individuals with delirium experience visual hallucinations over a brief time course and preferentially at night. Unlike people with schizophrenia, delirious patients also experience hallucinations with their eyes shut (Shea, 1998). Visual hallucinations in delirium are often composed of moving parts or geometric shapes, are poorly formed, and occur after a patient has already been noting visual distortion and illusions. That is not to say that people with schizophrenia don't have visual hallucinations of inanimate objects, shadows, bursts of color, or streaks of light, but this is less common than in delirium. Visual hallucinations in patients with schizophrenia are more likely to be crisp, occur in broad daylight, and include full-bodied figures of people who hold some importance to them. People with schizophrenia will also commonly hallucinate body parts, fantastic creatures, images with religious significance, or animals (Sadock, 2009). In schizophrenia spectrum disorders, the visual hallucination often occurs suddenly, without any warning, but within the context of, or accompanied by, other types of hallucinations. Unlike those experienced by people with schizophrenia, visual hallucinations in the delirious may be frightening or otherwise emotionally provocative, but they often have little personal significance to the patient (Shea, 1998). Due to this experience of salience, and like with auditory hallucinations, visual hallucinations in schizophrenia are often interpreted within a delusional construct.

Case Example

Joe is a 70-year-old white male, in good physical condition, who is well known to you and presents to your office for a routine medication-management session. Over the years, Joe has experienced periodic and vivid visual hallucinations. Today he tells you excitedly that, while watching a rerun of his favorite Western on television yesterday, he looked up and saw a crucified Jesus Christ in the corner of his living room. He described the image as being about eight feet tall and appearing much like religious images of Jesus he had seen in the past, but much more real. He insists that he must have seen Jesus just as he was 2,000 years ago when he was crucified, that Jesus had let him see the exact scene as it had occurred. He recalls that Jesus looked down on him and held his gaze, and he felt a reassuring warmth spread all over his body. He notes closing his eyes, and then opening them several times, with the image remaining before him. After several minutes, the image faded away, leaving Joe feeling content and renewed in his religious convictions.

Tactile, olfactory, and gustatory hallucinations also occur in schizophrenia and related psychotic disorders but are less common than their auditory and visual counterparts. The presence of these hallucinations may merit investigation into the possibility of causative neurological or medical etiologies. Of these, tactile hallucinations may be the most frequently observed. "Formication," or the feeling that bugs are crawling on or under one's skin, is often seen in substance-intoxication or withdrawal but can occur within schizophrenia. Some patients experience sensations of being sexually assaulted, feeling that their genitals and/or anus is being penetrated or otherwise injured. Patients may also complain of being shocked, burned, or stabbed, by seen or unseen entities. Still others will describe being inhabited by other beings, experiencing sensations of spirits or souls coming into their bodies. Patients, often with co-occurring delusions of being controlled by an outside entity, will sometimes feel their body being moved or otherwise physically compelled to act. Gustatory or olfactory hallucinations seem to be less appreciated in schizophrenia but do occur. Patients with these hallucinations may complain of unpleasant smells, like feces or garbage, or will experience odd tastes like blood or metal (Sadock, 2009).

Case Examples

Ed is a 45-year-old African American male with schizophrenia who chronically experiences formication. Although he has never seen any insects on his body, he struggles with the belief that that he is infested with some kind of bug. He complains that he can feel these bugs crawling under the skin of his legs and into his nares and anus. He shows you shallow excoriations on his legs, and there is evidence of scarring from years of excessive skin scratching.

Tom is a 40-year-old white male with a history of schizophrenia. He complains again of difficulty sleeping due to his enemies' continued sexual assaults on his person. Although he does not see them, he complains that they somehow, in a way he cannot understand, stab his penis and testicles repeatedly and throughout the night. He is vague in his descriptions of how this occurs but is insistent that it is painful and distressing.

Katie is a 35-year-old white female with a long history of schizophrenia. She tells you, in some anger, that her roommates have been spreading their feces on her clothing and other personal belongings. Although she has never witnessed them doing this, and cannot see any evidence of such tampering, she notes that she frequently smells fecal material on her belongings. She blames her roommates for this, as she believes that they do not like her and are trying to induce her to move.

Illusions and Other Perceptual Disturbances

Illusions, or the misinterpretation of external stimuli, are not uncommon in schizophrenia. While most people experience illusions to a varying degree, it is not uncommon to elicit illusions from people with schizophrenia during a mental status exam. People with schizophrenia may, for example, hear voices in the sound of running water or in the buzz of a refrigerator. They may also interpret a shadow as a person or perceive someone's moving face as slowly melting in front of them. They may hear others' animated conversation as being about a murder these people committed. Just as in the case of hallucinations, people with schizophrenia may interpret these illusions as being salient and having a deep significance for them.

Feelings of "derealization" and depersonalization, while often considered pathognomonic for dissociative disorders or post-traumatic stress disorder (PTSD), can and do occur within many other mental, neurological, and medical disorders, including schizophrenia spectrum disorders (Shea, 1998). Patients with derealization symptoms will describe feeling as though something is unreal or dreamlike about their external environment. Derealization can classically be observed in delusional mood, where patients on the cusp of a psychotic break will sense that something inexplicable has changed in the world around them, triggering further development of delusional explanations. Depersonalization, or the feeling that one is disconnected from one's thoughts, feelings, and actions, can also occur in schizophrenia.

Case Example

James is a 55-year-old Asian male with a long history of schizophrenia. He notes chronic feelings that he lives in an unreal world, and that everything has a dreamlike and flat quality to it. He feels emotionally unconnected, and he experiences the world and the people in it as lacking in emotional depth. Sometimes these experiences are more intense than others, but he notes that, overall, this experience has persisted for years. He explains that this experience is a product of having been removed from his world and placed in an alternate reality by an alien race decades ago. He suspects that his family, friends, and psychiatric treatment team are merely alien depictions of human life within this alternate universe. He states that the feelings of unnaturalness can be unsettling.

Delusions

Delusions are classically considered to be fixed, false beliefs that do not change, even when evidence contradicting their validity is presented. The presence of delusions in schizophrenia is very common, with up to 70% of people with schizophrenia experiencing clinically significant delusions at some point during their illness. People with schizophrenia often have multiple delusions, and while some delusions can be quite immutable, others abate with reality testing or specific psychotherapeutic modalities (e.g., cognitive behavioral therapy [CBT]). Some loosely held delusions can be adequately addressed by simple reassurance. Still others dissipate over time without formal treatment intervention. It is not uncommon, though, for new delusions to seemingly "take the place" of former delusions. Complex, systematized delusions are most frequently observed in middle-aged patients, and these in particular can be a challenge to effectively treat (Sadock, 2009).

Historically, delusions were considered to develop over time, starting with a "soft sign," or potential herald, of psychosis—the presence of the previously mentioned delusional mood. In the evolution of delusions, delusional mood progresses to delusional perception. This is the perception of normal sensations as quite intense, and having (heretofore nonexistent) deep personal significance for the sufferer. Patients with delusional perceptions may also begin experiencing ideas of reference, which are thoughts that inconsequential events or coincidences potentially contain significant meaning for them. In other words, these events seem to have abnormal salience: they focus the sufferer's attention and end up driving cognitions and ensuing behaviors (Kapur, 2003). For individuals with ideas of reference, casual conversations between passengers on a bus, for example, may seem to pertain specifically to them. Songs on the radio, topics on news programs, or specific blog articles will seem directed to them. A burnt-out lamppost may seem especially notable, as can a cellphone heard ringing in a doctor's pocket. When these experiences are examined, including with the help of a therapist or psychiatrist, the person with ideas of reference is able to reality test, admitting that they may be mistaken as to the importance of the experience in question. When, on the other hand, the person maintains the importance of the referential experience, and when they become incorporated into new or preexisting delusional beliefs, ideas of reference become delusions of reference. This shift is seen when the patient transitions into having frank delusions, the final stage of the evolution of the delusional process. It should be noted here, again, that hallucinatory phenomena may fuel delusional constructs, with patient's formulating delusional ideas to make sense of their experience of hallucinations (Sadock, 2009).

Overvalued ideas can be conceptualized as an attenuated form of, or on one side of the spectrum of, delusions. An "overvalued idea" is an unreasonable belief or idea held by a person, but in contrast to a delusion, the person does not hold it in strong conviction (American Psychiatric Association, 2013). Overvalued ideas are not uncommon in the general population, and like ideas of reference, they are generally responsive to reality testing. An example could be a friend frequently discussing how he will write "The Great American Novel," even though he has no experience with writing and has invested no time or energy in doing so.

Delusions can be classified into one of many subtypes, as summarized in Table 1.2. Persecutory delusions are the most common type of delusion in schizophrenia spectrum disorders, followed by grandiose delusions. Historically, clinicians have

Table 1.2 Types of Delusions

Types of Delusions Included in DSM-5

Persecutory [Sometimes Called Paranoid] Delusions	Beliefs that one is being persecuted by an individual, group of individuals, or an organization, and involving fear of being harmed physically, mentally, and/or emotionally. Delusions of persecution may also revolve around believing that one's reputation or financial status is under attack.
	Examples: A patient has delusions that their neighbors are actively conspiring to have them evicted from their apartment, that the CIA is tracking the patient with the plan of eventually torturing them for information, or that an alien race is working to make the patient a sexual slave.

(continued)

Table 1.2 Continued

Grandiose Delusions	Involve the sufferer believing that they are powerful, famous, and/or extremely wealthy. Examples: A patient believes that he was once a famous basketball player or is the heir to a significant fortune.
Jealous [Sometimes Called "Othello Syndrome"] Delusions	Involves the strong belief, with no evidence, that one's romantic or sexual partner is being unfaithful. Examples: Believing that one's wife is sneaking out in the middle of the night to have sex with other people or that one's husband has contracted a sexually transmitted disease.
Erotomanic [Sometimes Called de Clérambault Delusions] Delusions	The belief that a stranger, who is often famous or otherwise high status, is in love with the sufferer. Examples: A patient believes that her former employer, with whom she had minimal contact, is in love with her and sends her songs on the radio to remind her of his devotion. A man sends multiple romantic letters, which sometimes are disturbing in their intensity and context, to his state representative, who, he maintains, sends him signals to increase his letter writing in her campaign commercials.
Somatic Delusions	The belief that there is something wrong with one's bodily functions and involving bodily sensations. Example: Patients with somatic delusions may believe that they have parasitic infestations or that their gastrointestinal system no longer functions.

Table 1.2 Continued

Mixed Delusions	Delusions that have features of more than one delusional type, with no type predominating.
Unspecified Delusions	The type of delusion cannot be determined or is not included in DSM-5 types.

Other Types of Delusions

Religious Delusions	Beliefs that may have grandiose and/or persecutory themes and concern religion or spiritual matters.
	Examples: A patient believes that he has been possessed by demons or that he is Moses.
Delusions of Control	The belief that one's body, part of one's body, or mind is being controlled by an external entity.
	Related Delusions or Passivity Phenomena:
	Thought insertion: the belief that thoughts foreign to one's own have been inserted into one's mind.
	Thought withdrawal: the belief that one's own thoughts have been pulled from one's mind by an external entity.
	Thought broadcasting: belief that one's thoughts can be heard or otherwise experienced by everyone, often in a passive way.
	Delusions of one's mind being read: belief that others are actively able to read one's thoughts and do so intentionally.
	Examples: A patient believes that his hands is compelled to move by an outside force, or that his thoughts can be controlled through an implanted chip.

(continued)

Table 1.2 Continued

Delusions of Sin or Guilt	Beliefs by the sufferer that they have committed a serious crime or are responsible for a bad outcome to which they could not possibly be connected. These patients often feel the need to be severely punished for perceived misdeeds and have intense feelings of guilt.
	Examples: A patient believes he was responsible for a murder to which he had no connection and so confesses to police. A patient is distressed in believing that she caused a devastating hurricane.
Nihilistic Delusions	A belief by the sufferer that they do not exist, or that part of their body does not exist. They may also believe that others don't exist. Finally, they may also maintain that the world around them is to be destroyed or has already been destroyed.
	Related Delusions:
	Cotard's syndrome: the sufferer believes that their organs or blood have been lost, or that they are dead.
	Capgras syndrome: the delusional belief that a person familiar to the sufferer has been replaced by an imposter.
	Related Delusions:
	Fregoli's syndrome: the belief that familiar people (or persecutors) can take the form of strangers.
	Intermetamorphosis: The belief that familiar persons can change their forms into that of another person.
	Examples: A patient with Cotard's syndrome refuses to eat, insisting that they don't have a stomach or intestines. A patient with Capgras syndrome is concerned that her parents have been replaced by Doppelgangers.

also been interested in whether or not a delusion is bizarre. Delusions are considered bizarre when they are extraordinary, incomprehensible, or impossible. Delusions of control, or feeling that one's body is being controlled by outside forces, are classic examples of bizarre delusions. In previous versions of the DSM, including DSM-IV-TR, the presence of bizarre delusions, even in the absence of other symptoms, would meet Category A criteria for diagnosis of schizophrenia. This convention has been dropped from DSM-5, as interrater reliability in determining whether or not a delusion is bizarre is moderate at best. It should also be noted that when subthreshold symptoms are present for delusions, the term "ideation" can often be used to describe a patients' thought content, e.g., paranoid ideation, grandiose ideation, or jealous ideation.

Disorganization Symptoms

Disorganized Speech

Disorganized speech is the final, core "positive symptom" in the DSM-5 Criterion A for schizophrenia. Along with either delusions or hallucinations, it must be present to make a diagnosis of schizophrenia. Speech disorganization is extremely important in the diagnosis of schizophrenia in that it reflects the thought-process disorganization indicative of formal thought disorder. Formal thought disorder is not uncommonly held to be pathognomonic of schizophrenia, and many experts consider it to have the greatest morbidity of all the symptoms associated with schizophrenia.

Conceptualizing disorganized speech as a positive symptom of schizophrenia is somewhat awkward, as there are positive and negative elements of thought process disorganization. Positive elements of thought process disorganization include intrusion of unrelated or bizarre thoughts into speech, and negative elements include poverty of thought associated with *alogia*, or lack of speech (Rule, 2005). Alogia is sometimes classified as a negative symptom of schizophrenia. Thought-process disorganization, further unlike the other positive symptoms of hallucinations and delusions, does not respond particularly well to treatment. Its presence is associated with earlier illness onset, and like with negative symptoms, is predictive of a worse illness course.

The DSM-5 specifically mentions "frequent derailment or incoherence" in illustrating disorganized speech. Incoherence indicates the presence of frankly unintelligible speech. Phrases like "word salad" or "glossolalia" are often used interchangeably in labeling incoherent speech. "Verbigeration" is closely related and used to describe speech in which words and phrases are repeated senselessly. Odd word usage, including neologisms (new words) that convey meaning only to the patient, and word approximations, for example calling a snow ski a "sled skate," are also common. "Clanging" is less common in schizophrenia but is classically associated with the disorder, and it describes speech in which words are connected by sounds rather than coherent ideas. Rhyming and alliteration are common in clanging; for example, "I have a craving. I crave carrots, cabbage, crabbage, canola oil, boil, toil, trouble, tracks!"

Derailment indicates a sudden change in the direction of speech, like a train derailing from its tracks and ending up in a destination different from the one intended. This is slightly different than thought blocking, also observed in schizophrenia, in which thought seems to come to a screeching halt. Patients with thought blocking describe feeling as though the thoughts simply left their heads. Concepts related to derailment include tangentiality and circumstantiality. Both are commonly noted in the mental status examination of patients with schizophrenia. When a patient is tangential, he/she will not answer your question. The patient may start out on topic but will end up speaking to a different point, or points, entirely. In circumstantiality, the patient will "talk around" the question, sometimes for an extended period, but will eventually return to provide an answer. Loosening of associations is like an extreme form of tangentiality, in which the patient shifts from one topic to another with minimal to no connections between topics. Extreme forms of loosening can lead to word salad, verbigeration, and general incoherence as described. While a mild loosening of associations can be seen with anxiety, in severe forms, it is a good indicator of schizophrenia spectrum disorder.

While disordered thinking and resultant disorganization of speech increase during acute exacerbation of illness, its presence can be noted in up to 50% of stable patients (Sadock, 2009), probably reflecting the underlying cognitive deficits of schizophrenia. These cognitive deficits are often at least mildly or moderately impairing at a person's baseline and affect multiple cognitive domains. Deficits are often seen in comprehension, attention, semantic organization, and fluency and complexity of speech. Patients may also have deficits in social cognition and will have difficulty recognizing social cues and modulating their behaviors to social situations. Problems with working memory and poor executive functioning are also common, as is anosognosia, or lack of insight. Anosognosia is a particular problem for many people with schizophrenia, with some practitioners estimating that over half of the patients with this disorder have moderate to severe impairment in their awareness of having a mental disorder (Amador et al., 1994). Some patients with severe anosognosia will maintain that they do not have an illness and will persistently refuse treatment. Others may agree that they have an illness but still lack insight into their need for treatment. Still others may reject their diagnosis but appreciate the importance of treatment. These patients, for example, may recognize that antipsychotics help quiet "voices," but do not believe that they have a mental illness. Anosognosia often persists for patients over time, to varying degrees, but it can fluctuate with the course of the illness.

Grossly Disorganized or Catatonic Behavior

The next DSM criterion for schizophrenia is disorganized behavior. Like disorganized speech, this symptom is often classified as a positive one, although it is not considered a "core" positive symptom. Persons with schizophrenia with grossly disorganized behavior may have episodes of seemingly unprovoked physical or verbal aggression, which can lead to the patients' harming themselves or others. Perhaps more commonly, they will experience difficulties in caring for themselves. Such individuals may struggle with activities of daily living, including obtaining adequate nutrition and dressing themselves. They may, for instance, present to clinic in the middle of summer, in dire need of a bath, and wearing several layers of non-matching and ill-fitting winter clothing. They may also present with low BMI's or have concerning cigarette burns on their pants. It is also worth noting that these individuals may have particular trouble taking their prescribed medication, including for serious medical illness like hypertension or diabetes.

Historically, people with schizophrenia who had profound symptoms of disorganization were classified as having *hebephrenia*. Aside from disorganized behavior, the patients with hebephrenia frequently manifested inappropriate affect. So, too, can today's patients with grossly disorganized behavior, appearing quite angry or irritable without any internal or external stimulus. They may also appear rather silly and laugh inappropriately.

These odd affects can also be reflected in speech prosody, which can be childlike or vacuous. Disorganization of motor behavior may be subtle or, in the case of catatonia, quite extreme. Odd and repetitive movements are core features of disorganized motor behavior. Examples include patients' rocking, shaking or wringing their hands, and pulling at their hair or limbs. Patients may pace, absently turn pages in an upside-down book or magazine, or repeatedly attempt to pull firmly fixed signs off the walls of an inpatient unit. Sometimes these disorganized movements are quite complex, and patients appear as if engaging in some invisible but recognizable physical task, like directing an orchestra. If performed repeatedly and in a ritualistic way, these disorganized behaviors might be classified as *stereotypy*. If the movements are mimicries of others' movements, they are classified as *echopraxia*. An important consideration when evaluating possible motor disorganization would be to rule out extrapyramidal symptoms, like akathisia in individuals who pace and fidget, and tardive dyskinesia in those with repetitive movements, particularly when they appear involuntary.

Catatonia is defined, per the DSM-5, as "a marked decrease in reactivity to the environment." It can be seen in schizophrenia, mood disorders, and medical conditions. Overall, it is diagnosed less frequently in schizophrenia, at least in United States and Europe, than it once was, possibly as a result of antipsychotic treatment. Catatonia is often associated with seemingly purposeless movements, many of which will appear stereotyped. When the movements are excessive and continuous, catatonic excitement is said to occur. On the opposite end of the catatonic spectrum, patients can become motionless, even stuporous, or maintain rigid postures for extended periods of time. Some of the postures are bizarre; for example, standing on one foot in the middle of the room or lying in bed with arms widespread. These patients will often exhibit other signs of profound negativism, resisting all instructions, and will be mute on exam. Other patients may repeat what is told to them and thus display echolalia. Others patients will have catalepsy, also called "waxy flexibility" (not to be confused with cataplexy). In catalepsy, patients hold the postures that others, often examiners, place them into for long periods of time. Echopraxia, or the mimicry of others' movements, can also be seen. Patients who recover from catatonia often have difficulty describing it, either not remembering it much at all or recalling it only vaguely. They may note having felt that they were not in control of their bodies at the time, stating that they were aware of what was going on around them but were unable to engage in any significant way.

Case Examples

Aniyan is a 43-year-old male from West Africa with schizophrenia. He tells you he had at least one episode of catatonia prior to his successful immigration to the United States. Aniyan reports that his mother had him put in a large hospital once, where he resided for well over a year, because he would not move or speak for long periods of time. He notes vague recollections of lying in bed, soaked in urine, and feeling that he could not move his body or communicate with anyone. He is not sure how this episode resolved, but he says he eventually left the hospital on antipsychotic medications and moved back to his village.

Bao is a 50-year-old Vietnamese male who recently moved to the United States. You are called to see him on the unit, as staff are concerned that he is maintaining "yoga" postures for long time periods. When you see Bao, he is standing hunched over, arms widespread, and staring vacantly into space. He is mute, and he does not seem to engage with you in any way. He does not move when you ask him to sit down. His arms are rigid when you gingerly attempt an exam. Suddenly, he leaps backwards, striking his body on a wall and then slowly slumping to the ground. He smiles oddly and does not appear to be in any pain.

Negative Symptoms

"Negative symptoms" can be conceptualized as a lack, or deficit, in emotion, thought, or behavior. Classically, we often think of negative symptoms as a legacy of Bleulerian thought. Students are frequently taught Bleuler's rubric of "The Four A's" of schizophrenia: *association, affect, autism,* and *ambivalence.* Negative symptoms remain important in the diagnosis of schizophrenia, with diminished emotional expression, seen on exam as blunting or flattening of affect or diminished speech prosody (intonation), being highlighted by the DSM-5. Also emphasized in these diagnostic criteria is "avolition," or a decrease in purposeful, self-motivated and initiated activities. These two symptoms have been conceptualized as encompassing of other traditional negative symptoms, illustrated in Table 1.3.

Other, traditional negative symptoms seem better classified in other domains or symptom clusters. These are summarized in Table 1.4 for the sake of thoroughness.

Negative symptoms can occur across the schizophrenia spectrum of illnesses. In schizophrenia, however, their burden is often profound and heavily associated with morbidity. Negative symptoms are clinically challenging to treat, especially as they don't seem to respond much, if at all, to antipsychotic medications. Patients with significant and primarily negative symptoms during stable periods, as well as during periods of decompensation, have been described as having "deficit syndrome." It has been estimated that 15% of individuals newly diagnosed with schizophrenia would meet proposed criteria for deficit syndrome, as would a quarter or more of more established patients (Kirkpatrick et al., 2001).

Negative symptoms can only be deemed primary, or caused by schizophrenia, by exclusion. "Secondary negativism" encompasses seemingly negative symptoms actually caused by medication side effects, positive symptoms of schizophrenia, depressive symptoms, or other etiologies. For example, patients who appear asocial may have persecutory delusions or strong paranoid ideations that lead them to isolate from others. Social stigma and limited opportunities for social interactions can also mimic asociality. Anhedonia can be seen during episodes of depression, which are not uncommon in people with schizophrenia. Extrapyramidal symptoms, like the affective flattening and bradykinesia seen with drug-induced Parkinsonism, can also be confused with avolition (Peralta et al., 2000).

Mood and Anxiety Symptoms

Although not included in the diagnostic criteria for the disorder, many experts agree that disturbances in mood and clinically significant anxiety are exceedingly common in people with schizophrenia. Recognition and treatment of these major mental health comorbidities is essential. While their toll on the lives of people with schizophrenia is not well studied or understood, poorly controlled anxiety and mood symptoms may increase the severity of psychotic symptoms, contribute to substance use, and, in the extreme cases, can place the patient at greater risk for violence towards self or others (Sadock, 2009).

Table 1.3 Negative Symptoms

Diminished emotional expression	Includes affective flattening (e.g., blunted, or in the extreme flat, affect) and diminished speech prosody.
Avolition	Represents a decrease in purposeful, self-motivated, and self-initiated activities. It also includes symptoms of anhedonia (decreased ability to experience pleasure) and asociality (apparent lack of interest in social activity).

People with schizophrenia can have manic and depressive episodes. This is worth expressly stating, as confusion abounded with previous editions of the DSM relating to the diagnostic criteria of "schizoaffective disorder." Some clinicians considered an episode of mania or depression in a patient meeting diagnostic criteria for schizophrenia to be indicative of the presence of schizoaffective disorder. This led to overdiagnosis of schizoaffective disorder. DSM-5 criteria clarify that patients who meet Criterion A for schizophrenia can be diagnosed with schizoaffective disorder if a major mood episode is present for the majority of the duration of the illness, when the illness is not effectively treated (including treatment resistance), is inadequately treated, or is untreated. The "majority of the duration of illness" means that symptoms must be present, not only in active periods of

Table 1.4 Negative Symptoms Better Classified into Disorganization and/or Cognitive Domains

Poverty of speech/alogia

Inappropriate affect (e.g., patient laughs incessantly without apparent internal or external stimuli)

Attentional impairment

Social cognition deficits, including the ability to perceive, interpret, and act in accordance to the intentions or actions of other people illness, but in residual periods as well. As such, patients with schizophrenia can have episodes of mania or depression in the course of their illness without meeting diagnostic criteria for schizoaffective disorder.

Mania can be difficult to tease out from acute psychotic exacerbation, but it presents in schizophrenia much in the same way as it does in bipolar disorder. Its hallmark continues to be expansive, irritable, or elevated mood with increased energy and/or activity. Depression in schizophrenia is very common, and it is likely that most people with schizophrenia have had at least one episode of depression (meeting full criteria for major depression). Sub-syndromal episodes of depression arguably occur in most individuals with schizophrenia. Episodes of depression in schizophrenia can occur during acute psychotic decompensation and resolve when psychosis abates, or they can occur during otherwise more stable periods of schizophrenia. Much attention has been paid to post-psychotic depression, or the depression that arises during recovery from a psychotic episode. Post-psychotic depression has been linked to patients' having increasing insight into the severity and chronicity of schizophrenia, leading to much psychic distress at the risk of future decompensations and possible disability. Post-psychotic depression should be aggressively treated, as it unsurprisingly presents an increased risk of suicide (Fenton, 2000).

Patients with schizophrenia and depression give histories significant for feeling subjectively depressed, worthless, or inappropriately guilty, and they may also have recurring thoughts of death and/or suicidal ideation. Other classical symptoms of depression, including anhedonia, psychomotor disturbances, cognitive complaints, and disturbances in sleep and appetite, can sometimes be difficult to tease apart from preexisting symptoms of schizophrenia or side effects from antipsychotic medications. For example, psychomotor slowing seen in depression may mimic akinesia caused by high-dose typical antipsychotics. Akinesia can present with or without other symptoms of Parkinsonism. Some controversy also exists as to whether antipsychotics can, in rare cases, lead to dysphoria, but this claim has been largely contested (Mulholland & Coopers, 2000).

Generalized anxiety disorder is not uncommon in people with schizophrenia, with a prevalence estimated at around 11% (Achim, Maziade, Raymond, Olivier, Merette, & Roy, 2011). Social phobia, which can be difficult to tease out from paranoid ideations, negative symptoms, and deficits in social cognition, occurs in 15–40% of patients (Sadock, 2009). Panic attacks and panic disorder are also relatively common in schizophrenia, with an estimated 25% prevalence of panic attacks in this population and a 15% prevalence of panic disorder (Buckley, Miller, Lehrer, & Castle, 2009). Panic disorder may be related to worse outcomes in schizophrenia spectrum disorders and has been associated with overall more severe illness. Panic attacks have been clinically observed to occur more frequently in patients with paranoid ideations (Sadock, 2009).

While some symptoms of PTSD can raise concern for a psychotic spectrum disorder, thus causing confusion in differential diagnosis, there does appear to be a large comorbidity of PTSD in schizophrenia. Among those with schizophrenia, the prevalence of PTSD has been estimated at 29% (Buckley, Miller, Lehrer, & Castle, 2009). Trauma, particularly childhood trauma, has long been recognized as a risk factor for the development of schizophrenia, and PTSD has been found, in some patients, to be antecedent to first-episode schizophrenia. Persons with schizophrenia more frequently develop PTSD during the course of their illness. People with schizophrenia are not infrequently victims of crime, largely due to social and environmental factors, and can be seen as "easy marks" by criminals. Treatment, particularly forced medications or seclusion and restraint, can also be experienced as extremely traumatic to psychotic patients. As such, these interventions must be used as a last resort, with careful consideration of patient preference and patient perception of the proposed intervention.

Up to a third of people with schizophrenia have comorbid obsessive-compulsive disorder (OCD) (Sadock, 2009). The symptoms of OCD can mimic psychotic symptoms, and severe obsessions can be difficult to tease out from delusions, particularly in individuals with OCD with poor insight. When present in schizophrenia, obsessive compulsive symptoms appear much like those in people with OCD. Some of these symptoms, though, may be incorporated into patient's hallucinations or delusions; e.g., a patient with known schizophrenia who hears voices telling him to wash his hands repeatedly, which he then does compulsively. The presence of OCD in schizophrenia does seem to be linked to worse outcomes than for just schizophrenia alone (Poyurovsky, Weizman, & Weizman, 2004).

The presence of obsessive-compulsive symptoms (OCS) in the prodrome of first-episode schizophrenia has long been of research interest, as there may be overlap in the neurobiology of OCD and schizophrenia. Sometimes OCS fade as psychotic symptoms progress, but they often persist. Some have theorized about the presence of a unique "schizo-obsessive" disorder, although evidence supporting this is mixed (Bottas, Cooke, & Richter, 2005). Interestingly, there also exists a higher prevalence of OCS in patients on certain antipsychotic medications, particularly clozapine, than in patients not on any, or on other, antipsychotic medications (Scheltema, Swets, Machielsen, & Korver, 2012). This correlation is poorly understood and could be related to iatrogenic treatment effect or underlying illness characteristics, particularly as Clozaril is generally reserved for treatment-resistant individuals. Clozaril may, for example, treat severe psychotic symptoms so well that previously masked OCS symptoms can then be seen clinically.

Suicide

Suicide is a significant cause of excess mortality in schizophrenia. It is commonly taught that 10% of people with schizophrenia successfully complete suicide, which is probably based on the findings of a 1977 review (Miles, 1977) and a few long-term follow-up studies. This rate has been challenged in recent years, with concerns about the statistical modelling used in these older works. Suicide rate in schizophrenia may be closer to 5% (Palmer, Pankratz, & Bostwick, 2005), although the lifetime prevalence of suicide attempts is still much higher, ranging from 20–40% (Pompili et al., 2007). Risk for suicide in schizophrenia seems to be highest early in the course of illness and around the time of hospitalization or discharge. Having insight into one's illness and fear of further mental deterioration may be risk factors. Prominent persecutory delusions, high premorbid functioning, and post-psychotic depression are significant risks for suicide. Other general risk factors for suicide, including substance use, hopelessness, family stressors, social isolation, agitation, and being young, white, male, and unmarried, also increase the risk of suicide in someone with schizophrenia. It is thought that people with schizophrenia who attempt suicide may utilize more lethal means, have a stronger intention to die, and tend to make multiple attempts (Pompili et al., 2007).

Case Example

A 24-year-old white male, recently diagnosed with schizophrenia, presents to your outpatient clinic after being discharged from the hospital two weeks ago, where he had received intensive treatment for nearly two months for auditory hallucinations, persecutory delusions, and agitation. On interview, the patient currently denies any positive symptoms of psychosis. He reports that he is currently on leave from his doctoral program in chemistry, and he believes he may have to drop out. The patient states that he believes that he will never be able to finish school, let alone pursue his dreams of becoming a professor. The patient also admits that he recently broke up with his longtime girlfriend. He confides to you, "I love her, and I just can't keep putting her through this." He has also withdrawn from his family, partially because he remains angry at his father for committing him to the hospital, even though he agrees that he was ill and in need of treatment. The patient does report medication adherence, but he admits to drinking two or three neat whiskeys every night "just to relax." You suspect that he is depressed. He refuses more intensive treatment: "I just got out of the hospital. I need some space. I'll come back and see you about med refills in a few weeks." He denies any suicidal ideation, planning, or acts of furtherance. He denies access to weapons. He is ambivalent about starting an antidepressant and ultimately refuses this, appearing somewhat frustrated with you. "I know you're just trying to help, but you and I both know that schizophrenia ruins lives. I guess I'm just going to have to accept that." Two weeks later, you receive a tearful call from his ex-girlfriend, alerting you that the patient was found dead in his apartment of an apparently self-inflicted gunshot wound.

Violence

Violence in schizophrenia is a controversial topic. Patients, caregivers, and the mental health community at large are rightly concerned about the sensationalization of violence committed by people with schizophrenia, as this increases the societal stigma against this already marginalized group. People with schizophrenia, in fact, are more likely to be victims than perpetrators of violent crime, and less than 10% of societal violence is attributable to people with schizophrenia (Walsh et al., 2002). Most violent acts perpetrated by people with schizophrenia will also be carried out against caregivers, friends, or mental health workers, especially during the course of attempts to modify patients' behavior.

Risk factors for violence in schizophrenia include traditional risk factors for violence, including male gender and a previous history of violent acts. Traditionally, the presence of persecutory delusions has been thought to increase violence, although recent evidence casts this into some doubt (Walsh et al., 2002). In addition, while clinicians are attuned to the presence of command auditory hallucinations in traditional violence assessments, it is not clear that they present a significant risk factor for violence, at least in isolation from other risk factors (Monahan et al., 2000). Comorbid antisocial personality disorder or childhood conduct disorder do appear to be risk factors for violence perpetration (Sadock, 2009). Substance misuse particularly increases risk of violence in people with schizophrenia. Some argue that the presence of substance abuse is responsible for most of the excess risk of violence in people with schizophrenia (Fazel et al., 2009). Most agree, though, that nonadherence with psychiatric treatment, particularly with prescribed medications, might be the greatest risk factor for violence in this group.

Schizoaffective Disorder

"Schizoaffective disorder" is an attempt to classify patients who don't neatly fit the Kraepelinian dichotomy of serious mental illness, in which patients either have primary affective or psychotic disorders. Schizoaffective disorder has long been held to have more in common with schizophrenia than with mood disorders, and the phenomenology of schizoaffective disorder greatly overlaps with that of schizophrenia. It is likely for this reason that many studies of schizophrenia include people with schizoaffective disorder as subjects.

Schizoaffective disorder is thought to be much less common than schizophrenia, and as such, it should be diagnosed sparingly. There was much concern about over-diagnosis in the recent past, at least partially stemming from the diagnostic criteria of previous editions of the DSM. DSM-5 attempts to limit the use of the schizoaffective diagnosis to a very specific group of patients, rather than its being applied, for example, to anyone with schizophrenia who has had a major mood episode. While DSM-5 specifies that symptoms meeting criteria for a major mood episode must be present for at least 50% of the course of the illness, including both active and residual periods, there remains confusion about the effects of treatment. Some authors note that episodes that require treatment with an antidepressant or mood-stabilizing agent, and subsequent failure to successfully discontinue such treatment would be equivalent to the patient having prominent mood symptoms.

Some question schizoaffective disorder's diagnostic validity and reliability as a diagnosis altogether (Maier, 2006); therefore, many proposed that it not be included in DSM-5. Phenomenological concerns largely stem from issues with the original Kraepelinian dichotomy, given that episodes of mania and depression are frequently observed in patients with schizophrenia. An additional diagnostic concern is the stability of the schizoaffective diagnosis. Some people diagnosed with schizoaffective disorder will go on to be diagnosed with schizophrenia once seemingly prominent mood episodes become less pronounced in the overall course of the illness (Malaspina et al., 2013).

In addition to the mood episodes as described, to meet diagnostic criteria for schizoaffective disorder in the DSM-5, patients must essentially meet the other criteria for schizophrenia, except for impairment in occupational functioning. People with schizoaffective disorder may not manifest significant impairment in this domain, although they can have the negative, disorganized, and/ or cognitive symptoms commonly found in people with schizophrenia. There is some evidence, though, that these symptoms may be more attenuated in people with schizoaffective disorder, and traditionally, schizoaffective disorder was often considered to have a better outcome than schizophrenia (Harrow, Grossman, Herbener, & Davies, 2000). Suicide risk and associated risk factors are considered to be about the same as for schizophrenia, and rates and manifestations of comorbidity with anxiety and substance disorders are similar to schizophrenia as well.

Delusional Disorder

Delusional disorders were once called "paranoid disorders," or simply "paranoia," and they have been recognized since ancient times. Kraepelin wrote about paranoia as a distinct form of psychotic illness, and like some earlier writers, described the disorder as consisting of non-bizarre and well-developed delusions (Sadock, 2009). Importantly, in this disorder, cognition and personality were thought to go undisturbed. The DSM-IV diagnosis of delusional disorders did not stray much from this traditional framework, with criteria emphasizing non-bizarre delusions, minimal hallucinatory experiences, and no significant functional deterioration. Behaviors should neither be bizarre or odd, outside of the scope of the impact of the delusion. Hallucinations, too, must center on the delusional theme and not be prominent. The patient may realize that his or her beliefs seem farfetched or unrealistic, but their insight is often quite poor. Mood episodes, particularly depression (but including mania) can occur in delusional disorder, but like with schizophrenia, their duration must be brief in relation to the majority of the illness.

Case Example

The patient is a 40-year-old white female who is a bank teller, has a boyfriend, and attends church weekly. She also has a long history of persecutory delusions, chiefly that her neighbors want her to move from her apartment. She has complained, for at least the last five years, that the neighbors collect and leave dog feces in her yard, pour water on her doorstep when it could freeze, and are tampering with her mail. The patient also reports she hears the neighbors' voices through the apartment walls at times, conversing about their next move in their systematic plot to make her leave the complex. Today, she notes frustration with her seeming inability to audiotape these conversations. She shows you multiple pictures on her cell phone that she has collected to support her assertions about the mail tampering, but they don't seem to show anything of significance. The patient reaffirms that she largely avoids the neighbors as she remains frightened of them, but she has told her landlord about her concerns multiple times. She notes that he again tried to reassure her that no one wants her to move. The patient states that she is trying hard not to discuss these concerns with her boyfriend, as she worries that "he'll think I'm crazy if I keep talking about it." Her last boyfriend broke up with her, "because he was tired of hearing about it." Towards the end of your session today, she proudly tells you she recently won an award at work for exemplary customer service. At the same time, she laughs that she's still looking forward to her upcoming vacation. She has plans to travel to see an old friend who lives out of state.

The DSM-5 conceptualization of delusional disorder marks a very slight change in course from previous editions of the DSM. Chiefly, bizarre delusions are no longer exclusionary in diagnosing delusional disorder. The DSM-5 also clarifies that mental disorders including body dysmorphic disorder or obsessive compulsive disorder cannot better account for the disturbance. These disorders in particular can present with absent insight or delusional beliefs to the extent that the presence of a delusional disorder will often come into question. For example, someone with obsessive compulsive disorder may firmly believe that if they don't check the lock on their door seven times, their house will be broken into by an intruder. A patient with body dysmorphic disorder may absolutely believe that they have a misshapen ear despite much reassurance to the contrary. Neither of these patients would qualify for a diagnosis of delusional disorder, as their symptoms can be attributed to their underlying psychiatric disorder.

Persecutory delusions are the most common types of delusions in delusional disorder. Other DSM-5 subtypes include *erotomanic, grandiose, jealous, somatic, mixed* (no one delusional theme is prominent), and *unspecified* types (cannot be determined or not included in the criteria). Further explanation and illustration of these delusional types can be found in the "Delusions and Halluciantions" section of "Schizophrenia" in this chapter. It should be noted that the diagnosis of "delusional disorder" is generally stable over time, but a subgroup of people with delusional disorder do seem to go on to develop schizophrenia.

It should be noted that "shared delusional disorder," often called *folie à deux*, was a diagnostic category in previous editions of the DSM. Diagnostic criteria for shared delusional disorders generally held that a primary person would instill delusional beliefs in secondary parties, and that these "secondaries" would be generally free of other psychiatric disorders. Over the years, many questions have arisen as to the validity of this underlying framework, with secondaries often being found to meet criteria for mental disorder on comprehensive evaluation. They also tend to require extensive treatment (Arnone, Patel, & Tan, 2006). In DSM-5, shared delusional disorders are not represented as a separate diagnostic category. If two or more people share a delusion, and each affected party meets criteria for a delusional disorder, each person is said to have delusional disorder. If the delusional beliefs are shared, but full criteria for delusional disorder in one party are not quite met, then for that person, "other specified schizophrenia spectrum and other psychotic disorder" can be used as a diagnosis.

Brief Psychotic Disorder

Brief psychotic disorders are, by definition, brief, and they have a sudden onset. The brevity of the disorder is in stark contrast to the often chronic course of schizophrenia. Brief psychotic disorder also lacks the prodromal period of symptoms that usually precedes schizophrenia. They are relatively rare and seem to occur more often in women (Susser & Wanderling, 1994). There may also be a higher prevalence for brief psychotic disorders in developing countries (Susser & Wanderling, 1994). It may be linked to culture-bound syndromes. For example, the *bouffée délirante* of West Africa and Haiti might be classifiable as a brief psychotic disorder, and its symptoms include hallucinations, paranoid ideations and/or delusions, confusion, and psychomotor agitation. It is often preceded by concerns about witchcraft or other magical persecution. In Europe, diagnoses such as "amentia" and "cycloid psychosis" have been used to describe time-limited psychoses (the latter with periodic reoccurrences) with good outcomes. As such, these diagnoses appear similar to brief psychotic disorder.

   People who experience a brief psychotic disorder often feel emotionally overwhelmed or confused and may need intensive care, including hospitalization, to ensure that their basic needs are being met. There is, additionally, an increased risk for suicidal behavior, so this should be monitored for as well. Risk factors for this disorder include, per the DSM-5, "traits in the psychoticism domain," which would include suspiciousness, negative affectivity, and perceptual dysregulation. Individuals with personality disorders or traits, particularly those that fall in the Cluster A (e.g., schizotypal, paranoid) or Cluster B (e.g., borderline personality disorder) categories, seem more likely to develop this disorder as well. It should be noted that individuals with personality disorders do experience transient periods of psychotic symptoms, usually in the face of psychosocial stressors, but these usually last less than a day. If the symptoms persist for longer than that, a diagnosis of brief psychotic disorder should be considered.

Research into brief psychotic disorder is rather limited. Much of the work in this area has been done with subjects meeting criteria for the *International Statistical Classification of Diseases and Related Health Problems, 10th Edition* (ICD-10) "acute and transient psychotic disorders," which does not map neatly onto the DSM-5 diagnosis of brief psychotic disorders. The ICD-10 diagnosis is less specific and includes individuals who, by DSM criteria, would be diagnosed as having schizophreniform disorder or unspecified schizophrenia spectrum and other psychotic disorders.

Brief psychotic disorders can also be diagnostically challenging. They can be difficult to differentiate from substance/medication-induced psychotic disorder and from psychotic disorder due to another medical condition. It is, furthermore, a diagnosis that cannot be definitively given until symptoms have resolved, so as to ensure that the illness did not exceed the prescribed time course. Brief psychotic disorders can also carry the specifier "with postpartum onset" if the symptoms occur during pregnancy or within four weeks postpartum. Most episodes of postpartum psychoses, though, are largely attributable to other, more chronic, mental health disorders. Postpartum psychoses are identified as brief psychotic disorders only if the new mother does not have another underlying psychotic or mood disorder, such as schizophrenia (25% risk of puerperal, psychotic exacerbation) (Sit et al., 2006) or bipolar disorder (20–30% occurrence of postpartum psychosis) (Jones & Craddock, 2001). It is generally thought that most episodes of postpartum psychoses are attributable to bipolar disorders (Sit, Rothschild, & Wisner, 2006).

Case Example

Jane is a 24-year-old Latina with no premorbid psychiatric history who was brought to the emergency room by her fiancé shortly after her brother's funeral. During the funeral, Jane threw herself onto her brother's coffin, screaming that he was alive and that her family must open the coffin. The patient's father managed to remove her from the coffin, after which time she ran out into a busy street, where she was nearly struck by a car. The fiancé then insisted she have a medical evaluation.

In the emergency department, Jane continues to weep loudly and scream that her brother is not dead, that "they are burying him alive!" She seems confused and disoriented and is surprised when she is told she's in an emergency room. Per her fiancé's report, since shortly after hearing of her brother's death three days ago, Jane has been weeping for much of the day. Her fiancé also reports that she appears to be intermittently agitated, pacing and wringing her hands, and has refused to eat and is not sleeping. He notes that she often seems distracted and will not talk to anyone when addressed. The fiancé states that he has caught her repeatedly mumbling to herself and, on one occasion, she told him that she could hear "the voices of the angels." He insists that she does not use drugs or alcohol. You decide to admit Jane to the hospital for inability to care for herself. Her medical work-up is benign, and toxicology reports are negative. During her hospitalization, she is maintained on PRN Risperdal for psychotic symptoms. Within the week, the patient has returned to her baseline and is discharged home on no scheduled medications.

Schizophreniform Disorder

While its historical diagnostic criteria were broader in scope, in recent decades, "schizophreniform disorder" has been relegated to the status of a variant of schizophrenia, a sort of brief schizophrenia that lasts at least one month but less than six months. As such, the symptoms of schizophreniform disorder are essentially identical to those of schizophrenia, and schizophreniform disorder is often associated with first-episode schizophrenia as it has a high conversion rate to this disorder.

Classically, schizophreniform disorder was thought not only to be brief in course but to also have a sudden onset. The modern DSM, in contrast, accounts for prodromal symptoms as part of the illness time course, allowing for a more gradual onset of symptoms. Like with brief psychotic disorder, due to its short duration, it can be difficult to differentiate schizophreniform disorder from a substance or medication-induced psychotic disorder and from psychotic disorder due to another medical condition. It can also be a challenge to tease apart from other mental disorders, particularly schizophrenia, as establishing a clear time course of symptoms can be difficult, particularly if the patient has received successful treatment. Again like with brief psychotic disorder, schizophreniform disorder can only be diagnosed definitively after symptom resolution, and it can only be diagnosed provisionally (if it must be diagnosed) during its active course.

The DSM-5 notes that up to a third of individuals diagnosed as having schizophreniform disorders will recover. Most individuals diagnosed with schizophreniform disorder, however, appear to convert to other illnesses later. At two years, the McLean-Harvard International First-Episode Project found that the diagnosis of schizophreniform disorder held up in only 10.5% of cases (Salvatore et al., 2009). Most studies show that 45–75% of patients convert to schizophrenia or schizoaffective disorders (Sadock, 2009), with DSM-5 noting that two-thirds of patients generally convert to schizophrenia or schizoaffective disorder. A smaller number, probably less than 15%, will go on to be diagnosed with a mood disorder (Sadock, 2009). This conversion to mood disorder is more likely to occur in patients who had been diagnosed with schizophreniform disorder with good prognostic features, a DSM specifier. This group is also more likely to retain their original schizophreniform diagnosis. To meet criteria for "good prognostic features," a patient must manifest at least two of several signs or symptoms, including no affective blunting or flattening and "confusion and perplexity." If disturbances in behaviors or functioning occur, it is considered a good prognostic indicator if this occurs within four weeks of symptom onset. Good premorbid functioning is also considered to be a predictor of a better prognosis.

Schizotypal Personality Disorder

Schizotypal personality disorder is unique in that it is classified by the DSM-5 both as a personality disorder and as part of the schizophrenia spectrum of disorders. It seems to have some genetic basis and is more common among relatives of patients with schizophrenia. Like other personality disorders, it represents a stable and enduring set of traits that usually manifest by adolescence, leading to social and/or occupational impairment. People with schizotypal personality disorder are often viewed by others as eccentric due to their odd behaviors, beliefs, style of dress, and patterns of speech reflecting thought-process disturbance. People with schizotypal personality disorder may exhibit magical thinking and manifest beliefs in, for example, supernatural or paranormal phenomena that differ from subcultural norms. They may have ideas of reference and bodily illusions, and like with other personality disorders, it is not uncommon for individuals with this disorder to experience transient psychotic episodes. These episodes are self-limited, last no more than a few hours, and generally occur in the context of increased stress. Also as is not uncommon with other personality disorders, persons with schizotypal personality disorder experience difficulty in making and keeping relationships. They generally desire friendships but may come across as being uninterested in intimacy and closeness. Paranoid ideations and pervasive suspiciousness can prevent individuals with schizoptypal personality disorder from initiating gestures of friendship, and their odd affects and difficulty with social cues and reciprocity can keep potential friends at bay. Social stigma attached to being perceived as eccentric also affects their ability to form relationships, and people with schizotypal personality disorder are often well attuned to others' perceptions of their differentness.

Most people diagnosed with schizotypal personality disorder maintain this diagnosis over time and do not convert to other psychotic spectrum disorders. They are not likely to seek treatment for the disorder itself. They may accept care for comorbid conditions, particularly anxiety and depression, which are probably as common in schizotypal personality disorder as they are in other disorders in the schizophrenia spectrum. It is also not uncommon for schizotypal personality disorder to co-occur with other personality disorders.

Case Example

Marianne is a 60-year-old white female who lives alone in a small apartment in a quiet area of the city. She makes money selling homemade items online, as she has always had difficulties in keeping an "office job." She has no close friends. She has two sisters, one with schizophrenia, with whom she has occasional contact. She is not sure where her other sister lives. Her landlord finds her to be a reliable tenant, if a bit messy and odd in her dress and behaviors. Marianne frequently wears long, flowing garments that she has collected over the years, many of which are torn and covered in tea stains, and she attaches little bells to them as she thinks the ringing attracts fairy folk.

She will occasionally attempt conversation with the employees in the post office, with whom she regularly interacts to ship her wares, but the more she tries, the more she feels ill at ease. The postal workers are kindly to her, but they find her flat affect and stilted speech to be a little unsettling, and they chuckle with each other about her appearance. Marianne picks up on their discomfort, and it bothers her a great deal. She will occasionally vent on blogs about how lonely she is, and how difficult it is to be different, but her writing rarely elicits much comment, as it is so hard to follow.

Concluding Thoughts

Schizophrenia spectrum disorders have a complex phenomenology and a history that is as rich as it is indefinite. As the phenomenology of schizophrenia became increasingly appreciated, perhaps with the rise of the disorder itself, the diagnostic criteria became more precise. From ancient accounts of madness to the medieval writings of Ibn Sina, from the early studies of Pinel to the seminal works of Kraepelin, scholars through the ages have worked to understand and classify the symptoms of severe mental illness. In the modern era of the Feighner Criteria and the subsequent Diagnostic and Statistical Manuals, the diagnostic criteria for schizophrenia spectrum disorders, and the phenomenology that helped inform it, have allowed clinicians and their patients alike to identify and label the disorder with increasing consistency. While essential to modern psychiatric treatment, diagnosis and phenomenological classifications alone must not be considered sufficient to understand any one patient's illness. Working to appreciate an individual's experience of illness, to hear their own unique story, is the cornerstone of successful treatment of any disorder, schizophrenia spectrum disorders notwithstanding.

Self-Learning Questions

1. Schizophrenia might be:
    a. a disorder that has afflicted people since ancient times
    b. an illness that arose in the seventeenth or eighteenth century
    c. an illness whose defining features are a product of culture and time
    d. any of the above

2. Emil Kraepelin:
    a. has been called the father of biological psychiatry and the modern nosological approach to psychiatric illnesses
    b. is associated with the "4 A's" of schizophrenia (autism, loosening of associations, ambivalence, and affective incongruence)
    c. wrote about First-Rank Symptoms
    d. is a leader in the Anti-Psychiatry Movement

3. Positive symptoms of schizophrenia include:
    a. hallucinations
    b. delusions
    c. anhedonia
    d. social cognitive deficits
    e. both a and b

4. Negative symptoms are not found in:
    a. schizophrenia
    b. schizoaffective disorder
    c. delusional disorder
    d. none of the above

5. Patients struggling with disorganization symptoms may experience problems with
    a. hygiene and general self care
    b. sudden and seemingly unprovoked acts of aggression or self harm
    c. odd and repetitive movements
    d. all of the above

6. When considering the presence of possible negative symptoms, important rule-outs include
   a. side effects of medication
   b. positive symptoms affecting social functioning
   c. depressive symptoms
   d. social stigma
   e. all of the above

Key Learning Points

- The concept of schizophrenia as a medical illness took root in the late nineteenth century, but psychotic spectrum disorders, in some form, have existed for far longer.
- Emil Kraepelin, Eugen Bleuler, and Kurt Schneider were instrumental in the early understanding of schizophrenia and helped give rise to modern diagnostic efforts.
- Spurred on by criticism from the Anti-Psychiatry Movement, and utilizing the Feighner Criteria, the American Psychiatric Association has continued to hone and better define schizophrenia as a diagnosis in successive editions of the *Diagnostic and Statistical Manual*.
- Phenomenology is the study of both signs and symptoms as well as patients' subjective experiences of a disorder. An understanding of phenomenology helps us provide patient-centered care.
- Common symptoms of schizophrenia spectrum disorders include perceptual disturbances (most commonly auditory hallucinations), delusions, disorganization of speech and behavior, and negative symptoms. Mood and anxiety symptoms are also common.

References

Achim, A. M., Maziade, M., Raymond, É., Olivier, D., Mérette, C., & Roy, M. A. (2011). How prevalent are anxiety disorders in schizophrenia? A meta-analysis and critical review on a significant association. *Schizophrenia Bulletin*, *37*(4), 811–821.

Amador, X. F., Flaum, M., Andreasen, N. C., Strauss, D. H., Yale, S. A., Clark, S. C., et al. (1994). Awareness of illness in schizophrenia and schizoaffective and mood disorders. *Archives of General Psychiatry*, *51*(10), 826–836.

American Psychiatric Association. (1968). *Diagnostic and Statistical Manual of Mental Disorders, Second Edition*. Washington, D.C.: American Psychiatric Association.

American Psychiatric Association. (2013). *Diagnostic and Statistical Manual of Mental Disorders, Fifth Edition*. Arlington, VA: American Psychiatric Association.

Arnone, D., Patel, A., & Tan, G. M. Y. (2006). The nosological significance of folie à deux: A review of the literature. *Annals of General Psychiatry*, *5*(1), 1–8.

Bottas, A., Cooke, R. G., & Richter, M. A. (2005). Comorbidity and pathophysiology of obsessive-compulsive disorder in schizophrenia: Is there evidence for a schizo-obsessive subtype of schizophrenia? *Journal of Psychiatry and Neuroscience*, *30*(3), 187–193.

Buckley, P. F., Miller, B. J., Lehrer, D. S., & Castle, D. J. (2009). Psychiatric comorbidities and schizophrenia. *Schizophrenia Bulletin*, *35*(2), 383–402.

Fazel, S., Gulati, G., Linsell, L., Geddes, J. R., & Grann, M. (2009). Schizophrenia and violence: Systematic review and meta-analysis. *PLoS Medicine*, *6*(8), e1000120.

Fenton, W. S. (2000). Depression, suicide, and suicide prevention in schizophrenia. *Suicide and Life-Threatening Behavior*, *30*(1), 34–49.

Fraguas, D., & Breathnach, C. S. (2009). Problems with retrospective studies of the presence of schizophrenia. *History of Psychiatry*, *20*(1), 61–71.

Harkavy-Friedman, J. M., Kimhy, D., Nelson, E. A., Venarde, D. F., Malaspina, D., & Mann, J. J. (2003). Suicide attempts in schizophrenia: The role of command auditory hallucinations for suicide. *Journal of Clinical Psychiatry*, *64*(8), 871–874.

Harrow, M., Grossman, L. S., Herbener, E. S., & Davies, E. W. (2000). Ten-year outcome: Patients with schizoaffective disorders, schizophrenia, affective disorders and mood-incongruent psychotic symptoms. *The British Journal of Psychiatry*, *177*(5), 421–426.

Hare, E. H. (1988). Schizophrenia as a recent disease. *British Journal of Psychiatry*, *153*, 521–531.

Jeste, D. V., Del Carmen, R., Lohr, J. B., & Wyatt, R. J. (1985). Did schizophrenia exist before the eighteenth century? *Comprehensive Psychiatry*, *26*(6), 493–503.

Jones, I., & Craddock, N. (2001). Familiality of the puerperal trigger in bipolar disorder: results of a family study. *American Journal of Psychiatry*, *158*(6), 913–917.

Kapur, S. (2003). Psychosis as a state of aberrant salience: A framework linking biology, phenomenology, and pharmacology in schizophrenia. *American Journal of Psychiatry*, *160*(1), 13–23.

Kirkpatrick, B., Buchanan, R. W., Ross, D. E., & Carpenter, W. T.Jr. (2001). A separate disease within the syndrome of schizophrenia. *Archives of General Psychiatry*, *58*(2), 165–171.

Maier, W. (2006). Do schizoaffective disorders exist at all? *Acta Psychiatrica Scandinavica*, *113*(5), 369–371.

Malaspina, D., Owen, M. J., Heckers, S., Tandon, R., Bustillo, J., Schultz, S., et al. (2013). Schizoaffective disorder in the DSM-5. *Schizophrenia Research*, *150*(1), 21–25.

McNiel, D. E., Eisner, J. P., & Binder, R. L. (2000). The relationship between command hallucinations and violence. *Psychiatric Services*, *51*(10), 1288–1292.

Monahan, J., Steadman, H. J., Robbins, P. C., Silver, E., Appelbaum, P. S., Grisso, T., et al. (2000). Developing a clinically useful actuarial tool for assessing violence risk. *The British Journal of Psychiatry*, *176*(4), 312–319.

Miles, C. P. (1977). Conditions predisposing to suicide: A review. *The Journal of Nervous and Mental Disease*, *164*(4), 231–246.

Mulholland, C., & Cooper, S. (2000). The symptom of depression in schizophrenia and its management. *Advances in Psychiatric Treatment*, *6*(3), 169–177.

Palmer, B. A., Pankratz, V. S., & Bostwick, J. M. (2005). The lifetime risk of suicide in schizophrenia: A reexamination. *Archives of General Psychiatry*, *62*(3), 247–253.

Peralta, V., Cuesta, M. J., Martinez-Larrea, A., & Serrano, J. F. (2000). Differentiating primary from secondary negative symptoms in schizophrenia: A study of neuroleptic-naïve patients before and after treatment. *American Journal of Psychiatry*, *157*(9), 1461–1466.

Pompili, M., Armador, X. F., Girardi, P., Harkavy-Friedman, J., Harrow, M., Kaplan, K., et al. (2007). Suicide risk in schizophrenia: Learning from the past to change the future. *Annals of General Psychiatry*, *6*, 10.

Poyurovsky, M., Weizman, A., & Weizman, R. (2004). Obsessive-compulsive disorder in schizophrenia. *Central Nervous System Drugs*, *18*(14), 989–1010.

Rule, A. (2005). Ordered thoughts on thought disorder. *Psychiatric Bulletin*, *29*(12), 462–464.

Sadock, B. J., Sadock, V.A., & Ruiz, P. (2009). *Comprehensive Textbook of Psychiatry, vols. 1 & 2*. Philadelphia, PA: Lippincott Williams & Wilkins.

Salvatore, P., Baldessarini, R. J., Tohen, M., Khalsa, H. M. K., Sanchez-Toledo, J. P., Zarate Jr, C. A., et al. (2009). The McLean-Harvard First Episode Project: Two-year stability of DSM-IV diagnoses in 500 first-episode psychotic disorder patients. *The Journal of Clinical Psychiatry*, *70*(4), 458.

Scheltema, B. A., Swets, M., Machielsen, M., & Korver, N. (2012). Obsessive-compulsive symptoms in patients with schizophrenia: A naturalistic cross-sectional study comparing treatment with clozapine, olanzapine, risperidone, and no antipsychotics in 543 patients. *The Journal of Clinical Psychiatry*, *73*(11), 1395–1402.

Shea, S. C. (1998). *Psychiatric Interviewing. The Art of Understanding*. Philadelphia, PA: Saunders.

Sit, D., Rothschild, A. J., & Wisner, K. L. (2006). A review of postpartum psychosis. *Journal of Women's Health*, *15*(4), 352–368.

Susser, E., & Wanderling, J. (1994). Epidemiology of nonaffective acute remitting psychosis vs schizophrenia: Sex and sociocultural setting. *Archives of General Psychiatry*, *51*(4), 294–301.

Teeple, R. C., Caplan, J. P., & Stern, T. A. (2009). Visual hallucinations: Differential diagnosis and treatment. *Primary Care Companion to the Journal of Clinical Psychiatry*, *11*(1), 26–32.

Walsh, E., Buchanan, A., & Fahy, T. (2002). Violence and schizophrenia: Examining the evidence. *The British Journal of Psychiatry*, *180*(6), 490–495.

Diagnosis and Assessment of Schizophrenia and Related Psychoses

Jason B. Rosenstock

Introduction and Overall Approach

Case Example

Darla is a 38-year-old African-American female who presents to the clinic because of recent "unusual experiences." She really didn't want to come, but her mom made her. Darla has been having trouble at work: her boss asked her to take a couple of days off because everyone's concerned about how she's been acting. Darla hasn't been concentrating lately, and her cubicle mate heard her talking to her computer screen, saying strange things about being monitored. Darla laughs it off, saying she's just frustrated that her employer blocks certain websites. But her mom has also noticed that Darla hasn't been herself lately, calling her at all hours of the night, concerned about sounds she's hearing in her house. Darla says the place seems to be "surrounded" by crickets, making these noises that disturb her. She's called exterminators to try to get rid of them, with no luck. "I'm not crazy," Darla insists, as she crosses her arms and glares at her mother.

You, as the provider, want to help Darla and her mom. To do that, you need to do your best to determine the diagnosis; that will predict the course and prognosis, and it will identify any possible treatment options. Even at this early point in Darla's history, you may be thinking about some sort of psychotic process. Could the sound of crickets be an auditory hallucination? Might delusions explain her beliefs about the computer?

But making a diagnosis of a psychotic disorder isn't easy. There's no blood test or brain scan that will clinch such a diagnosis. It takes time, careful attention to detail, good history-taking, an observant mental status examination, judicious use of tests, a pursuit of collateral sources of information, and longitudinal monitoring. As a provider, you need to be a bit of a detective in order to diagnose schizophrenia or other psychotic disorders.

And while you may think a psychotic disorder may be likely, many other conditions can produce psychotic symptoms, including other psychiatric disorders and other medical diseases. Could Darla have a brain tumor? Is she using substances? Or might she have no illness at all, other than stress, perhaps?

In this chapter, you'll find a framework for approaching patients like Darla, how to think about the assessment process for patients presenting with possible psychotic symptoms, and how to make (and share) a definitive diagnose that will inform future treatment. We will explore the components of the assessment, the differential diagnosis for psychosis, diagnostic criteria for psychotic disorders along with common comorbidities, and how this diagnosis can help with identification and management, especially for patients early in their illness.

Here are the *key summary points* to keep in mind as you approach patients:

- Assessment requires both detailed cross-sectional (mental status exam, interview) as well as longitudinal (history, course) components.
- Presentations may be heterogeneous, although diagnosis is grounded in key DSM-5 criteria, based on patient history and clinical assessment, not on labs or tests.
- Providers must rule out other psychiatric and medical conditions that can cause psychosis before settling on a primary psychotic disorder, although comorbidities are common.
- Take care when making a diagnosis of a psychotic disorder: it takes time, and when the news is delivered to patients and families, providers must be encouraging and hopeful about recovery.
- Early identification is crucial, because early treatment with specialized providers and using psychosis-specific biological and psychosocial interventions can significantly improve illness outcomes.

Let's explore each of these areas in more detail in the following sections.

Clinical Assessment

Case Example

Darla's symptoms have been continuing for several months, after she moved into her first house by herself. She denies depressive symptoms currently, although she has been depressed before, after being sexually assaulted in her teens. She denies using substances other than smoking "an occasional joint." Her medical history is significant for complex partial epilepsy; she still has several seizures per year, although she has had none for months, and she's on several antiepileptic medications. Her brother is in treatment for bipolar disorder; an aunt was "institutionalized" for years. Mental status exam is notable for an odd affect, inappropriate laughter at times, with some response latency and possible thought blocking. She's suspicious of what you're writing on your clipboard about her, and she seems distracted during the encounter. When you ask permission to talk to her neurologist, she refuses.

The assessment of patients presenting with possible psychotic symptoms parallels what you would do with any patient, with perhaps a few areas of special attention. You would perform a history, do a mental status examination, perform a physical examination (with a focus on neurological systems), order any indicated or screening laboratory tests, and consider standardized diagnostic tools such as neuropsychological testing or rating scales. And you would follow the patient over time to gather adequate data through history and serial assessments. All this will allow you to make an appropriate diagnosis.

Table 2.1 shows the components of the history, with notes about key areas of attention in psychosis.

Most of this history can come from the patient directly, although you will probably need to access collateral sources of information (family members, old medical records, other health providers, referral sources) to flesh out the detail and corroborate the patient's story. This process is not likely to be completed in one assessment visit but will require several contacts or visits over time.

The objective component of your assessment begins with the mental status examination (Table 2.2).

Table 2.1 Components of History

History Components	Psychosis-Specific Areas for Attention
Chief Complaint	Patients with psychosis more commonly are brought to clinical attention by others; they may lack insight or deny symptoms, so the chief complaint may frequently come from family members, employers, or other supports.
History of Present Illness	Obviously, the more detail you can obtain about the nature of the possible psychotic symptoms, the easier it will be to determine what they represent. Onset, duration, temporal connection with other associated symptoms, and functional effects are key data points here. Getting a person's "theory of illness" may be very useful as well.
Psychiatric History	Past illness/diagnoses, medications/therapies, hospitalizations, etc., provide context and help with the differential diagnosis and treatment planning. Antipsychotic usage would be a particular focus, along with aggressive and suicidal ideation/behavior.
Medical History	What other medical illnesses has the patient had, and how well controlled have they been lately? Prior head injury and seizure activity deserve special attention here, along with current medication usage. Don't forget about gynecological history. You may need to collaborate with other medical providers, so that information is useful, too.

(continued)

Table 2.1 Continued

History Components	Psychosis-Specific Areas for Attention
Family History	Obviously, any family history of psychotic symptoms/disorders increases the likelihood that the patient has a primary psychotic disorder (Maki et al., 2005). But other family medical conditions may yield possibilities for the differential diagnosis. And histories of metabolic syndrome conditions may help inform choice of treatment, down the road.
Social History	Pay special attention to birth and development here—were there obstetric complications or developmental delays? How did the patient do in school? What's their work history? Social relationships can clue you in to a variety of psychotic and related disorders. Other risk factors for schizophrenia include urban living, frequent housing moves or immigration during childhood, and traumatic life events.
Substance Use History	Current use is of course hugely important in the differential diagnosis, with substances like cannabis, stimulants, and hallucinogens of particular interest. Prior heavy cannabis use is also a risk factor for schizophrenia (Radhakrishnan et al., 2014).

Table 2.2 Mental Status Examination

Mental Status Exam Components	Psychosis-Specific Areas for Attention
Appearance/ Behavior	Personal grooming and self-care may be affected by psychosis; eye contact is often erratic. Patients may present guarded and suspicious, or resistant to assessment. Neuromotor findings can be seen even prior to treatment, including dyskinesias or "soft signs" like incoordination (Chan & Gottesman, 2008).
Mood/Affect	Significant mood findings may swing a differential diagnosis to non-psychotic conditions, although depressive symptoms are frequently seen in primary psychotic disorders, and affect is often blunted (or odd or incongruent).
Speech	Dysarthria or other abnormal findings could suggest other medical diagnoses. In acute psychosis, speech is often fast and productive, although flights of ideas may suggest mania as an alternative diagnosis.
Thought Process	Findings such as tangentiality, circumstantiality, loose associations, or neologisms may suggest formal thought disorder. Disorganization and illogic may be the only positive symptom findings for some individuals with schizophrenia. Thought blocking is another important finding to look for.
Thought Content	Delusions of all types may be seen: persecutory, somatic, jealous, imposter, etc. (although some, like grandiose or nihilistic, may suggest mood disorder). Care must be taken to separate overvalued ideas from true delusions: how fixed and firmly held is the thought? This may require "pushing" or challenging the patient carefully on how strongly they believe a thought to be true.

(continued)

Table 2.2 Continued

Mental Status Exam Components	Psychosis-Specific Areas for Attention
	Other classic findings in psychotic disorders are thought interference— either withdrawal, insertion, or monitoring (mind-reading). Ideas of reference (e.g., receiving messages from the television) are also common.
	Sometimes obsessions are confused with delusions; these need to be elicited carefully. Lethality/dangerous concerns are of course of paramount importance.
Perception	Dissociation, illusions, and hallucinations need to be carefully screened for. Remember to ask about common hallucinations, but also look for behavior that suggests the patient may be experiencing perceptual abnormalities (e.g., scanning the room, appearing distracted, talking to himself/herself).
Cognition/ Sensorium	Psychosis in the context of clouded sensorium might suggest delirium or another medical process. Patients with schizophrenia may be concrete or have gaps in intelligence. They may also have cognitive deficits (especially inattention and working-memory problems).
Insight/ Judgment	As noted, patients frequently lack awareness that they have a problem. Assessing judgment can help, obviously, with treatment and disposition decisions.

Mental status findings in these areas may require special screening questions to elicit. Delusions, for instance, may be spontaneously mentioned, but often patients will hide these thoughts out of embarrassment or fear. Screening questions for psychosis might include these:

- Do you have any thoughts that you're reluctant to share with folks because you think they may not understand?
- Have you been having any thoughts that have been particularly bothersome or frightening to you?
- Do you feel like people around you may be trying to hurt you in some way, or hurt those you care about? Have you had other concerns about your safety?
- Have you ever felt like you had any special powers or abilities that other people just don't have?
- Do you feel like anyone is "messing" or interfering with your thoughts in any way?
- Have you felt like you have a hard time keeping track of your thoughts? Do people seem to have a hard time following your train of thought?

Also, with delusions, you want to assess whether or not they are bizarre or non-bizarre, systematized or non-systematized, mood-congruent or incongruent. Although there is some disagreement about the clinical significance of bizarre delusions (Cermolacce et al., 2010), and DSM-5 has eliminated that as a unique criterion for schizophrenia, the other parameters can help with diagnosis (mood-congruent suggests a primary mood disorder) and prognosis (systematized delusions are harder to treat).

When eliciting data about hallucinations, you want to get as much detail as you can about the phenomenology of the experiences:

- What sensory modalities are affected? (auditory, visual, tactile, gustatory, olfactory).
- Are the auditory phenomena perceived as external (heard in the environment) or internal (inside the head)?
- Can the patient make out specific voices? If so, whose, and what are they saying?
- Do the voices ever tell the patient to do anything specific?
- Do the voices ever talk directly to or about the patient?
- Are the hallucinations associated with each other in any way?

- Can the patient recognize that these are hallucinations?
- Can the patient do anything to make the phenomena go away?

To continue the objective assessment of the patient, someone needs to perform a thorough physical examination. The goal, of course, is to screen for medical conditions that could present with psychosis. Although any system could be relevant (e.g., endocrine, pulmonary, rheumatological), the highest-yield part of the physical exam will be the neurological exam. A thorough search for lateralizing or focal findings can suggest the need for further tests or examinations to rule out underlying neurological illness.

Laboratory tests and radiological exams are common parts of standard assessments in medical settings. Of course, in the work-up of psychiatric symptoms, there may be less use for lab screening and imaging tests, unless there are clear findings from the history or physical exam that suggest the need for additional work-up. Based on the most common medical conditions, and which are the cheapest/easiest tests to get, here is one list of tests for individuals with new presentations of psychosis:

- Complete blood count with differential
- Electrolytes
- Thyroid-stimulating hormone (TSH) test
- Urine drug screen
- Renal function tests (BUN/creatinine)
- Liver function tests (LFTs)
- Lipid profile
- Pregnancy test

The last two listed are more relevant when considering treatment initiation/options, rather than in assisting with the differential diagnosis. Some might argue that LFTs similarly are more for treatment considerations; the results are probably unlikely to inform the differential.

Other tests may be added as indicated. For instance, someone with a history of head injury or right-sided weakness nerve may benefit from neuroimaging. A patient with a family history of autoimmune disease should probably be screened themselves. Intravenous drug use might suggest human immunodeficiency virus (HIV) screening.

Some have argued that individuals presenting with new-onset psychotic symptoms deserve to have neuroimaging to rule out structural findings, even in the absence of neurological findings on exam. However, the yield on such screening is so low, and the costs are so high (both financial and in terms of chance findings), that it seems unwarranted as part of routine evaluation (Albon et al., 2008).

There is much attention being paid to identifying "biomarkers" that may assist with the diagnosis of schizophrenia. For instance, abnormal gamma-band activity on electroencephalogram (EEG), certain genetic polymorphisms in the coding for dopamine receptors, and levels of inflammatory cytokines may all carry some risk for, or be altered in, schizophrenia. But until such tests can be evaluated further, there is not yet a clear role for them in routine clinical practice (Prata et al., 2014).

There may be a slightly more important role for neuropsychological testing in the assessment of patients with psychosis. Projective testing (e.g., the Thematic Apperception Test), personality testing (e.g., the Minnesota Multiphasic Personality Inventory [MMPI]), and executive functioning testing (e.g., Continuous Performance Test) may all help to some extent, in some patients. Cognitive assessment of attention and working memory may also be useful in selecting treatment and monitoring outcomes.

In standard medical care, approximately 70% of the data needed for diagnosis come from history, 20% from the physical exam, and the remaining 10% from tests. In the work-up of psychotic symptoms, the proportion is probably similar, with perhaps less weight given to labs/tests and more accorded to the other components. But history remains key in the evaluation of psychosis, and the focus should be there.

Differential Diagnosis of Psychotic Symptoms

Once you have obtained thorough data from your assessment, you can proceed to evaluate the patient for the most likely diagnosis. Figure 2.1 outlines an approach to the patient's symptoms that may aid in assigning a proper diagnosis.

First, consider whether the person's symptoms represent a "real" disorder: Is it clinically significant, for instance, or not that concerning to anyone? Some beliefs seem like delusions but are actually very consistent with the beliefs of specific cultural subgroups—for instance, Native Americans believe that the spirit of a departed loved one may inhabit animals or birds. Holding that belief should not "count" as a delusion, if you are a member of that cultural community. Determining whether a symptom is "real" also includes ferreting out possible feigned psychotic symptoms.

Next, consider secondary causes of psychosis, particularly substance-induced psychosis or psychosis secondary to a medical condition. Finally, if none of these other possibilities applies, narrow down the diagnosis to a primary psychotic disorder (e.g., schizophrenia) or some other primary psychiatric condition (e.g., depression).

These question points in the differential are crucial in order to avoid overdiagnosing individuals. Not all psychotic symptoms are in fact clinically significant. About 15% of "normal" people will experience hallucinations at some point in their lives, without functional consequences or significant distress (Beavan et al., 2011). In bereavement, for instance, individuals commonly hear the voice of the deceased in the aftermath of the death. Moreover, experiences that some would call psychotic may occur commonly in certain cultural subgroups and contexts (e.g., religious beliefs about reincarnation, or "speaking in tongues").

Another possible diagnosis for psychotic symptoms is malingering. Although this is uncommon, some individuals do feign hallucinations or other experiences in an effort to be admitted to a hospital, avoid work or unpleasant tasks, or for other reasons. Atypical presentations, unusual or inconsistent symptoms, comorbid antisocial personality ,or acute psychosocial stressors raise the possibility of malingering (although this diagnosis may be very hard to confirm).

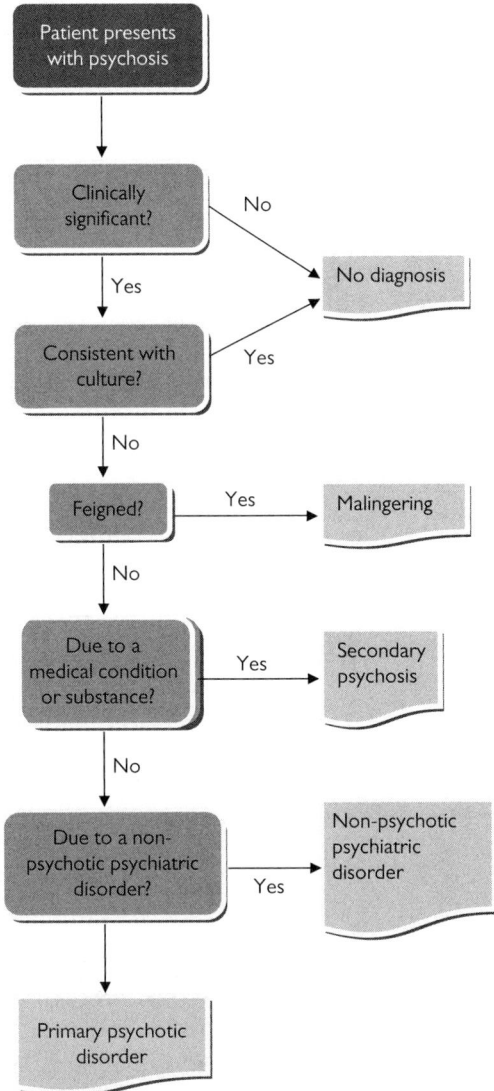

Figure 2.1 Assigning a diagnosis.

Assuming the psychotic symptoms are clinically significant, inconsistent with culture, and unfeigned, a provider should next consider secondary causes of psychosis. You want to rule out these causes first, because of course they require different treatments and are likely to have a different acuity.

Let us start with medical conditions that can cause psychosis. These conditions should move up on your differential diagnosis if:

- The symptoms represent a first episode of psychosis, particularly an early onset (under 15 years old) or a late onset (over 50 years old).
- There are uncommon or atypical features present (e.g., olfactory hallucinations).
- The patient has had a psychotic relapse after a long period of remission.
- Symptoms expressed differ substantially from prior episodes of psychosis.
- Neurological findings are noted on exam (e.g., lateralizing signs).
- The patient does not respond to standard treatments.

If you suspect a medical condition might be present, you should consider a variety of possibilities, which can be divided into neurological and other medical conditions (Table 2.3).

Table 2.3 Neurological Diseases That Can Produce Psychosis

Cerebrovascular	Stroke, vasculitis
Epilepsy	Complex partial (especially temporal lobe), absence
Movement Disorders	Huntington's, Parkinson's
Neoplastic	Brain tumor (especially frontal, limbic), paraneoplastic
Trauma	Concussion (especially left temporal), subdural hematomas
Autoimmune	Multiple sclerosis, lupus, anti–N-Methyl-D-Aspartate (NMDA) receptor encephalitis
Infectious	Herpes encephalitis, neurosyphilis, HIV, parasites, meningitis

Table 2.4 Non-Neurological Conditions That Can Produce Psychotic Symptoms

Endocrine	Thyroid (hyper/hypo), Cushing's, parathyroid, pheochromocytoma
Nutritional	B_{12}/folate/thiamine deficiency
Autoimmune	Systemic lupus erythematosus
Metabolic	Wilson's disease, acute intermittent porphyria, uremia
Medications	Anticholinergics, antihypertensives, steroids, disulfiram, etc.
Toxicities	Vitamins, lead, carbon monoxide, heavy metals

Non-neurological conditions to look out for include those listed in Table 2.4.

Reviewing the patient history while going over lists like this can prompt further work-up that may help identify a medical cause for symptoms.

The other secondary cause for psychotic symptoms is substance use. Providers often struggle to disentangle a person's psychosis from their substance use—there is often a temporal overlap, and many substances can cause symptoms identical to what might be seen in a primary psychotic disorder. Clinicians frequently misdiagnose patients in one or the other direction, and early in a person's course of illness, the diagnosis may change as new information is obtained or longitudinal follow-up reveals the most likely explanation for the patient's symptoms. Features such as a short duration of psychosis in the context of a lack of family history may suggest substance-induced psychotic disorder (Fiorentini et al., 2011).

Substance-induced psychosis can occur from a variety of substances, in either intoxicated or withdrawal states. The most common presentations are psychosis due to toxicity of stimulants (cocaine, amphetamines, methamphetamine) or hallucinogens (PCP ["angel dust"], LSD ["acid"], etc.). Cannabis, of course, is the most prevalent substance used in the general population (other than alcohol or nicotine), and it can produce both positive and negative symptoms that strongly resemble schizophrenia and related psychotic disorders. Even alcohol and sedative-hypnotics may be implicated, particularly in withdrawal states.

If you have eliminated secondary causes of the psychotic symptoms, you should turn your attention to other psychiatric conditions that may be responsible (Table 2.5). Psychotic symptoms like hallucinations and delusions can be features of

Table 2.5 Other Psychiatric Conditions That Can Produce Psychotic Symptoms

Disorder	Psychotic Symptoms
Depression/ Bipolar	Typically mood-congruent and temporally connected with mood episodes, not present when patients have a stable mood.
Borderline Personality	When stressed, patients with this condition may experience "micropsychosis"—usually brief, mild hallucinations or intense cognitive distortions that border on delusions.
Autism Spectrum	Such patients are frequently misdiagnosed with schizophrenia, although in autism the patients typically lack typical positive symptoms. They may be odd, socially isolated, with self-stimulating behaviors (such as self-talk) that cause misdiagnosis.
Post-Traumatic Stress	Individuals with trauma may have dissociation (e.g., flashbacks) that seems like psychosis; tactile hallucinations are not uncommon.
Major Neurocognitive	Delusions are often seen in dementia (patient misplaces things, becomes convinced that someone has stolen them), and hallucinations can be seen in delirium. Other cognitive and temporal features can serve to separate these from primary psychotic disorders.

a number of disorders in psychiatry, and features in the history and mental status can help decide which one may be present.

If all of these conditions have been ruled out, you can turn to primary psychotic disorders to see which diagnosis best fits the patient's pattern of symptoms and history.

Diagnostic Criteria for Schizophrenia and Related Psychoses

In the fifth edition of *The Diagnostic and Statistical Manual of Mental Disorders* (American Psychiatric Association, 2013), psychotic disorders have been classified as "schizophrenia spectrum and other psychotic disorders." Schizophrenia is the hallmark of this class, along with related conditions such as:

• schizoaffective disorder
• schizophreniform disorder
• brief psychotic disorder
• delusional disorder

Catatonia conditions are also included in the DSM-5 chapter on psychotic disorders, although this construct may be secondary to a variety of mental health and other medical conditions (not unique to psychosis); therefore, the DSM-5 has included catatonia as a specifier rather than as a separate diagnosis. Schizotypal personality disorder, on the other hand, is NOT included in this chapter, although it may in fact be a prodrome or precursor to schizophrenia in some individuals.

Schizotypal personality disorder (SPD) may be a good place to start when thinking about the differential diagnosis of possible psychosis. SPD is a condition that usually begins in adolescence, characterized by ongoing odd beliefs and speech, unusual perceptual experiences, and interpersonal deficits that affect functioning (Table 2.6). Patients with this condition may be particularly interested in concepts like astrology or mind-reading, when such concepts are not typically adhered to by the person's cultural group. They may experience unusual perceptual experiences such as illusions (e.g., interpreting the humming of the refrigerator as someone calling their name). They may also present as somewhat suspicious with inappropriate affect. SPD individuals, however, are not grossly psychotic: the odd beliefs do not reach delusional intensity, illusions do not become hallucinations, and most of these individuals will NOT go on to develop schizophrenia).

If the patient has clear psychotic symptoms such as loose associations, bizarre delusions, or frank hallucinations, then these symptoms are more severe than those typically seen in SPD, and the patient may have schizophrenia or one of the related psychotic disorders.

Schizophrenia is the most important of these disorders because of its prevalence, its functional consequences, its relevance

Table 2.6 Schizotypal Features

Thought content	Suspiciousness
	Referential ideas
	Odd beliefs
Perceptions	Illusions
Thought process	Mild disorganization
Affect	Blunted/inappropriate
Behavior	Odd/eccentric
Relationships	Few friends
	Social anxiety

Onset early in life, pervasive pattern, not due to a psychotic or other condition.

for translational neuroscience, and its response to treatment (Table 2.7). The diagnosis of schizophrenia depends on the identification of positive and negative symptoms lasting at least a month, causing significant functional decline over at least a six-month period of overall illness, with symptoms not caused by other conditions. This simple framework hides numerous complexities of diagnosis: distinguishing odd beliefs from delusions, for instance, or differentiating negative symptoms from depression, or deciding whether behavior is truly disorganized or simply odd, or even how long symptoms have actually lasted. This diagnostic approach also fails to address what many believe lies at the heart of schizophrenia—underlying cognitive deficits (e.g., in attention and working memory)—which have been deemed too non-specific to qualify as DSM-5 criteria. Despite the challenges, these criteria are fairly well operationalized and make it reasonably easy to make determination if a good history and mental status exam are obtained.

One of the key issues in diagnosing schizophrenia is its heterogeneity of presentation. Just two out of the five core positive and negative symptoms are required to make a diagnosis (at least one must be a positive symptom). That means that some individuals may have schizophrenia without having either delusions or hallucinations. There may be dozens of different combinations of symptom profiles that meet criteria for the illness.

Table 2.7 Schizophrenia Features

Positive Symptoms	Delusions
	Hallucinations
	Disorganized thought
	Disorganized behavior
Negative Symptoms	Flat affect, amotivation
Functioning	Social/occupational decline
Duration	1 month for core symptoms, 6 months' total duration
Rule-outs	Other psychosis/autism
	Other medical/substance

At least two positive/negative symptoms required.
Cognitive symptoms not included diagnostically.
Can specify first or multiple episodes, acute episode or in full or partial remission, with or without catatonia.

This approach recognizes that everyone with schizophrenia is a bit different, and that there are no pathognomonic signs or symptoms (not even hallucinations, which are the most commonly reported feature).

The DSM-5 criteria for schizophrenia are very similar to DSM-IV and older criteria sets. Previously, individuals could meet the core of "Criterion A" through the sole presence of either bizarre delusions or Schneiderian "First-Rank" symptoms (e.g., voices conversing about the person). These had been felt to be specific to schizophrenia, although recent evidence has cast doubt on that (Nordgaard et al., 2008); now, in DSM-5, individuals must have two full core symptoms to meet Criterion A.

Also, individuals with schizophrenia used to be diagnosed with a specific subtype of the illness—paranoid, disorganized, catatonic, undifferentiated, or residual. However, these subtypes were felt to be unstable and not that helpful for treatment or prognosis, so they have been eliminated (and replaced with a five-point dimensional severity indicator).

The other psychotic disorders are all related, based on symptom subtypes or duration of illness. If, for instance, the total illness duration has not yet reached six months (but exceeds one month), then *schizophreniform disorder* is the appropriate diagnosis to make. If the duration of symptoms is between one day and one month, than *brief psychotic disorder* would be the diagnosis. Neither condition requires significant functional decline. Brief psychotic disorder is often associated with a stressor of some sort.

In terms of symptom profiles, if the only psychotic symptom present is delusions, then *delusional disorder* may be the diagnosis (Table 2.8). For delusional disorder, the criteria are simple: one month or more of delusions without other significant psychotic symptoms (hallucinations, if present at all, must be mild and explicitly related to the delusions). Functional decline does not need to be present, and other conditions must be ruled out.

The other major symptom profile would be represented by *schizoaffective disorder*, a condition characterized by the longitudinal combination of psychotic symptoms with significant mood components. Controversy continues to swirl around this condition, with some questioning its validity (Heckers, 2009). There had been discussion that it might be eliminated in DSM-5; instead, criteria were clarified to make the classification easier to use. Specifically, patients must have:

- core symptoms of schizophrenia (one month or more of two or more psychotic symptoms, at least one positive);
- psychotic symptoms concurrent with a major mood episode (mania or depression);

Table 2.8 Delusional Disorder Features

Delusions	>1 month
	Any kind
	Bizarre/non-bizarre
	Hallucinations, if present at all, relate to delusions
Functioning	Minimal impairment
Rule-outs	Other mood/psychiatric
	Other medical/substance

Can specify first or multiple episodes, acute episode or in full or partial remission, with or without catatonia.

- psychotic symptoms for at least two weeks in the absence of mood symptoms;
- mood episodes present for more than 50% of the total duration of the illness.

And of course the symptoms cannot be due to other causes.

The algorithm in Figure 2.2 shows graphically how you might think about fitting these criteria sets to a specific patient scenario.

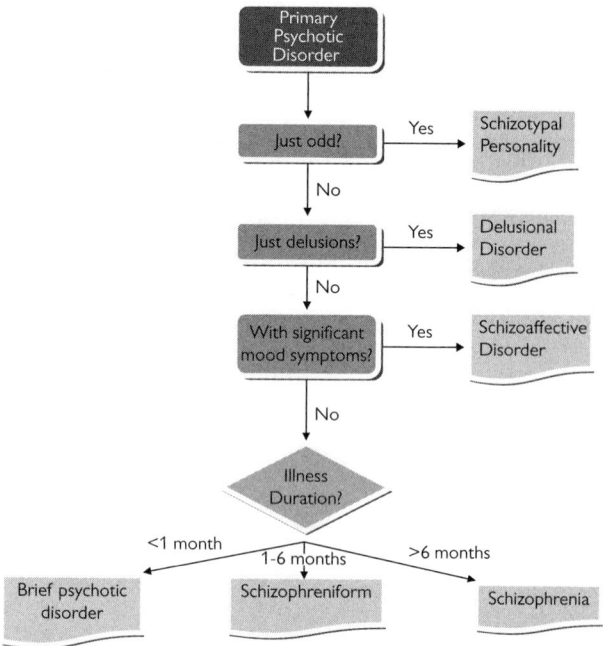

Figure 2.2 Fitting criteria sets to a specific case.

Comorbidity with Psychotic Disorders

People who have psychotic disorders may have other comorbid conditions (Buckley et al., 2009). These conditions may cloud the diagnosis or require additional treatment. Once a diagnosis of a psychotic disorder is made, providers should also be thinking about and screening for common comorbidities to insure that patients recover most fully.

Depression, for instance, is a key comorbidity, one that is often difficult to separate from core psychotic symptoms. Depressive symptoms are common in schizophrenia, and they may overlap with negative symptoms or deficit states (e.g., flat affect, low motivation, hypersomnia). Depressive symptoms can occur at the same time as positive psychotic symptoms, or they may follow a symptom flare (post-psychotic depression). As many as half of patients with schizophrenia will experience clinically significant depressive symptoms; such symptoms can dramatically impair quality of life and contribute to long-term risks such as suicide.

Mania can be part of schizoaffective disorder, although bipolar disorder is not typically a comorbid condition for other psychotic disorders. Some individuals with brief psychotic disorder or catatonic presentations may go on to develop mania/bipolar disorder.

Substance use is another common comorbidity. Anywhere from one-third to two-thirds of patients with psychotic disorders will misuse at least one substance, most commonly alcohol, cannabis, and cocaine (in that order). Nicotine, of course, is even more commonly used by patients with schizophrenia and schizoaffective disorder, a prevalence of perhaps 70–90%. Although the use of substances initially may raise the possibility of a secondary psychotic disorder (as outlined), more commonly individuals will have substance use in addition to a primary psychotic disorder—a variable temporal course that suggests two independently originating primary disorders, a true dual diagnosis.

Anxiety symptoms frequently develop in psychotic patients, and many carry a full anxiety disorder in addition to their primary psychotic disorder. Obsessive-compulsive disorder (OCD) or significant obsessive-compulsive symptoms may occur in one-third of patients, enough to make some observers describe a separate illness: schizo-obsessive disorder.

Other medical conditions are seen at higher rates among individuals with psychotic disorders, such as:

- metabolic syndrome
- pulmonary disease
- infectious disease
- epilepsy

Metabolic syndrome includes hypertension, hyperlipidemia, hyperglycemia, and obesity.

Incidence estimates vary widely, but it appears that as many as a third of individuals with psychotic disorders suffer from metabolic syndrome, a rate that increases with antipsychotic medication use; rates are much higher than in the general population, and this syndrome may be a large part of why individuals with severe and persistent mental illness have higher mortality than the general population (Mitchell et al., 2013).

Smoking rates may predispose individuals with psychotic disorders to higher rates of chronic obstructive pulmonary disease (COPD) than the general population. Patients are also more vulnerable to infectious diseases like tuberculosis, HIV, and viral hepatitis, a higher risk that may be related to lifestyle factors. The connection between epilepsy and psychotic disorders remains a mystery, but comorbidity rates have been consistently shown to be elevated (Casey et al., 2011).

Early Identification of Psychotic Disorders

A growing trend in schizophrenia research and treatment has been the increasing emphasis on early intervention as a way of improving outcome. Much evidence has accumulated that the duration of untreated psychosis is a strong predictor of ultimate outcome in schizophrenia, particularly remission rate and time to response (Dell'Osso et al., 2013). Furthermore, earlier interventions, with either psychotherapy or pharmacotherapy, may help reduce conversion rates in ultra-high-risk individuals from prodrome to full psychosis (Stafford et al., 2013). Although on one hand we want to be careful not to prematurely make a diagnosis of schizophrenia or early psychosis, on the other hand, the longer the wait to initiate treatment, the worse the outcome may be for the individual with symptoms.

Because of this conundrum and the difficulties in fully predicting who will develop full psychosis and who will not, most providers advocate very close monitoring for individuals who may be developing a psychotic disorder, and early intervention as soon as a diagnosis can be made. Several centers (e.g., Francey et al., 2010) have ongoing research programs designed to further explore risk factors and interventions for this population.

Giving the Diagnosis

It is difficult to make a diagnosis of schizophrenia or related psychotic disorder. But it is even harder to tell a patient or family about the diagnosis. Individuals fear the diagnosis, or have no idea about the implications. Some feel angry, sad, scared, or lost when they find out. And we as providers feel uncomfortable as we struggle to transmit confidence, expertise, and hope—even if we ourselves feel uncertain, ambivalent, and nervous.

Few training programs provide formal instruction on how to present the diagnosis of schizophrenia. Yet this is a communication skill like any other, a skill that can be learned and that—if done well—can improve outcomes for patients and families. We recommend a series of steps that can make the process easier for everyone, outlined in Table 2.9.

In your discussion of the diagnosis, you should expect some typical questions, and plan ahead for how you want to answer them:

- What is schizophrenia?
- Why did this happen?
- Is there anything we could have done to prevent it?
- Are there any other possible diagnoses?
- Will he/she get better?
- Will he/she be able to function? [marry, work, live independently, have children]
- What kind of treatments will be needed?
- What should we tell friends/family?

Patients and family members may need other information that they will NOT ask about, but that you should provide anyway (see Box 2.1). You should absolutely inform them about community resources that will be instrumental in managing the illness, particularly education and support resources for family members. The most important of these resources is the National Alliance on Mental Illness (NAMI), an advocacy and education organization particularly useful for family members coming to terms with a new diagnosis. In some ways, the most important single thing a provider can do when presenting the diagnosis of schizophrenia is to refer a family to NAMI for ongoing help, support, and information.

Table 2.9 Presenting the Diagnosis

Step	Description
Be sure	Obviously, the basic prerequisite for the "diagnosis discussion" is that you have made a diagnosis. You do NOT want to have the discussion prematurely, before you have firmly come down on a clear diagnosis. Once you have a diagnosis clearly made, however, you don't want to wait long—it's time to tell the patient and family.
Take time	Presenting a diagnosis takes time. It's not something that can be rushed. You have to presume that patients and families will have many questions; they will want you to spend time with them on this key issue. Block out adequate time for this discussion (typically an hour, sometimes more).
Make space	You want to do this in person, in a quiet and safe space, where people can be free to communicate their deepest emotions and questions. You don't want to do this in the patient's hospital room, or in a common area, or at the nurses' station. Commandeer a group room, or the social worker's office off the unit, or somewhere where everyone can sit comfortably and see each other.
Be inclusive	Key providers and staff members should be there, particularly anyone the patient identifies as a close support (e.g., doctor, nurse, social worker, etc.). This includes family members (patient, parents, siblings, etc.) and other relevant support people, if involved (e.g., significant other). Having everyone present makes it hard to schedule such a meeting, but it's much better to share the experience rather than try to "catch people up" if they miss it.

(continued)

Table 2.9 Continued

Step	Description
Plan ahead	Presenting a diagnosis takes planning. Team members should think carefully about how to discuss the situation. There should be full agreement on the diagnosis, of course, but also in terms of the approach to the patient and family. You should think about common and likely questions and how you will respond to them in this case (e.g., "Could the marijuana be contributing?" or "Will he be able to finish law school?").
Designate roles	Someone from the team should be designated as the "lead" for the meeting; this responsibility should be clear and acknowledged. Other roles include presenting facts, answering questions, following up, and so forth.
Say what's what	In the actual meeting, after basic introductions and a discussion of the goals of the meeting, it's best to begin by restating the facts of the case: what is known, what has been done, what test results have shown, etc.
Say what it means	Then, explain to the patient/family what these facts actually mean: what are the implications of all this? Were ALL other possibilities ruled out? Is there anything that is still pending or possible? How do these facts support a particular diagnosis? Ultimately, you want to state as clearly and directly as possible what you think the diagnosis is. Furthermore, you want to extend this discussion to what the diagnosis means for the future. Will the patient require specialized treatment/services? If so, what kind? What are the prognosis and the recovery potential? What kind of supports will be helpful going forward? This is a long discussion, but you want to begin it here.

Table 2.9 Continued   81

Step	Description
Check their comprehension	Ask the patient/family if they understand what's been said, and if they have any questions. Try to answer as best you can, as honestly as you can.
Monitor emotions	Check out the emotional reactions of patient/family members. Try to assess what's going on; ask directly to check it out. For instance, you can say something like: "I know this is a lot to take in. How are you doing with this? Feeling overwhelmed?" Or, "It seems like you're pretty angry about this—can you tell me more about how you're feeling?" Empathize with and validate emotions.
Normalize	Validate the lived experience of the patient and family. Explain that their reactions are common, typical, and expected, and that they are not alone in struggling with this kind of situation.
Accept	Acceptance is often hard and can take a long time. Patients may reject the diagnosis (due, perhaps, to lack of insight), and family members may have doubts. You as the provider may feel helpless, angry, or uncertain. Just like patients and family members need to accept things, you as the provider also need to accept the situation as it is, as best as you all can.
Be real	Your being genuine and honest about the situation will be extremely helpful for patients and family members. The more "real" you can be, the more they will see you as a reasonable "partner" in the process or treatment, and the more they will trust you overall. Try not to be the "sage on the stage," the aloof expert. Be a collaborator, an ally, a listener, and a carer.

(continued)

Table 2.9 Continued

Step	Description
Inspire hope	The process of recovery begins with hope for the future. Too often, when patients and families receive a diagnosis, they feel discouraged and helpless. It's particularly important at this early stage to begin engagement around recovery, by inspiring those affected with hope for a brighter future. This is being real, by the way; the diagnosis isn't a "death sentence" for sufferers. It's a chronic illness, yes, but one that can be managed and controlled like any other.
Go forward	The presentation of the diagnosis is just the start of an overall treatment relationship, either with you or with your colleagues. This relationship may occur over a lifetime, and because of the implications, it's important to start off on the right foot. Towards the end of the diagnosis meeting, it's worthwhile trying to agree on "next steps"—when you will meet again, what needs to be done before then, what can reasonably be expected over time, etc. Planning and agreeing upon frequency and type of contact will make it easier for patients and family members to start a therapeutic relationship with you and your colleagues.

Box 2.1 Suggested Patient and Family Educational Materials

"What Is Schizophrenia?" (National Institute of Mental Health, accessed Jan. 4, 2016):

http://www.nimh.nih.gov/health/publications/schizophrenia/index.shtml

Schizophrenia Health Center (WebMD, accessed Jan. 4, 2016): http://www.webmd.com/schizophrenia/default.htm

Schizophrenia.com (accessed Jan. 4, 2016): http://schizophrenia.com/

National Alliance on Mental Illness (accessed Jan. 4, 2016): http://www.nami.org/

Amador, X., & Johanson, A.-L. (2010). *I Am Not Sick, I Don't Need Help! How to Help Someone with Mental Illness Accept Treatment* (New York: Vida Press).
Mueser, K. T., & Gingerich, S. (2006). *The Complete Family Guide to Schizophrenia: Helping Your Loved One Get the Most Out of Life* (New York: Guilford Press).
Torrey, E. F. (2013). *Surviving Schizophrenia: A Manual for Families, Consumers and Providers* (6th edition) (New York: HarperCollins).

Conclusion

When someone presents with psychotic symptoms, the provider must do a careful assessment in order to make an accurate diagnosis. Cross-sectional and longitudinal assessment should include obtaining a detailed history from the patient and collateral sources, doing a careful examination (mental status and physical exams), and considering relevant labs/tests. Once completed, a thoughtful differential diagnosis process can help identify the correct diagnosis, which needs to be carefully communicated to patients and families to insure appropriate and rapid treatment and begin a process of recovery.

Self-Learning Questions

1. When screening for psychosis, the BEST question to ask a patient would be:
   a. Are you having auditory hallucinations?
   b. You're not hearing voices, are you?
   c. Has your imagination been playing tricks on you lately?
   d. Did anything unusual happen to you today?

2. Which of the following would NOT be considered a typical, core symptom of schizophrenia?
   a. Delusions
   b. Disorganized thought
   c. Flashbacks
   d. Hallucinations

3. A 40-year-old single man was first hospitalized at age 23 for hallucinations, delusions of persecution, and disorganized thoughts. Since then, he has been unable to work or develop friendships, and he was hospitalized 13 times for psychiatric treatment. In the last 10 years, his hallucinations, delusions, and disorganized thought processes became less severe. However, during the last 10 years, his speech has become less spontaneous, the relatedness and modulation of his affect have diminished, his mood has become shallow, and he spends each day watching television and smoking. Of the following, the most likely diagnosis is
   a. Bipolar disorder
   b. Delusional disorder
   c. Schizoaffective disorder
   d. Schizophrenia
   e. Undifferentiated somatoform disorder

4. When presenting the diagnosis of schizophrenia to a patient and family members, which of the following tasks would be most important to focus on, to best be helpful?
   a. Cautioning about functional limitations
   b. Explaining diagnostic criteria
   c. Inspiring hope for recovery
   d. Reviewing test results

Key Learning Points

- The diagnosis of a primary psychotic disorder is made primarily by obtaining a good longitudinal clinical history and doing a careful mental status exam.
- Before diagnosing a psychotic disorder, other conditions must be ruled out. Depression, anxiety, substance use, and general medical conditions are commonly comorbid with psychotic disorders, and the presence of any of these can make diagnosis and treatment challenging.
- Psychotic disorders can be distinguished from each other through careful attention to the duration of illness, type of psychotic symptoms, and presence of associated symptoms (especially mood).
- Presenting a diagnosis to a patient/family requires careful planning but is essential, and if done well, can help instill hope for recovery.
- Early identification and appropriate treatment can improve long-term outcomes for individuals with psychotic disorders.

References

Albon, E., Tsourapas, A., et al. (2008). Structural neuroimaging in psychosis: A systematic review and economic evaluation. *Health Technology Assessment*, *12*, iii–iv, ix–163.

American Psychiatric Association. (2013). *Diagnostic and Statistical Manual of Mental Disorders* (5th ed.). Arlington, VA: American Psychiatric Publishing.

Beavan, V., Read J., & Cartwright, C. (2011). The prevalence of voice-hearers in the general population: A literature review. *Journal of Mental Health*, *20*, 281–292.

Buckley, P. F., Miller, B. J., et al. (2009). Psychiatric comorbidities and schizophrenia. *Schizophrenia Bulletin*, *35*, 383–402.

Casey, D. A., Rodriguez, M., et al. (2011). Schizophrenia: Medical illness, mortality, and aging. *International Journal of Psychiatry Medicine*, *41*, 245–251.

Cermolacce, M., Sass L., & Parnas J. (2010). What is bizarre in bizarre delusions? A critical review. *Schizophrenia Bulletin*, *36*, 667–679.

Chan, R. C., & Gottesman, I. I. (2008). Neurological soft signs as candidate endophenotypes for schizophrenia: A shooting star or a Northern star? *Neuroscience and Biobehavioral Reviews*, *32*, 957–971.

Dell'Osso, B., Glick, I. D., et al. (2013). Can long-term outcomes be improved by shortening the duration of untreated illness in psychiatric disorders? A conceptual framework. *Psychopathology*, *46*, 14–21.

Fiorentini, A., Volonteri, L. S., et al. (2011). Substance-induced psychosis: A critical review of the literature. *Current Drug Abuse Reviews*, *4*, 228–240.

Francey, S. M., Nelson, B., et al. (2010). Who needs antipsychotic medication in the earliest stages of psychosis? A reconsideration of benefits, risks, neurobiology and ethics in the era of early intervention. *Schizophrenia Research*, *119*, 1–10.

Heckers, S. (2009). Is schizoaffective disorder a useful diagnosis? *Current Psychiatry Reports*, *11*, 332–337.

Maki, P., Veijola, J., et al. (2005). Predictors of schizophrenia—a review. *British Medical Bulletin*, *73–74*, 1–15.

Mitchell, A. J., Vancampfort, D., et al. (2013). Prevalence of metabolic syndrome and metabolic abnormalities in schizophrenia and related disorders—a systematic review and meta-analysis. *Schizophrenia Bulletin*, *39*, 306–318.

Nordgaard, J., Arnfred, S. M., et al. (2008). The diagnostic status of first-rank symptoms. *Schizophrenia Bulletin*, *34*, 137–154.

Prata, D., Mechelli, A., Kapur, S. (2014). Clinically meaningful biomarkers for psychosis: A systematic and quantitative review. *Neuroscience and Biobehavioral Reviews*, *45C*, 134–141.

Radhakrishnan, R., Wilkinson, S. T., D'Souza, D. C. (2014). Gone to pot—A review of the association between cannabis and psychosis. *Frontiers in Psychiatry*, *5*, 54.

Stafford, M. R., Jackson, H., et al. (2013). Early interventions to prevent psychosis: Systematic review and meta-analysis. *British Medical Journal*, *346*, f185.

Epidemiology
of Schizophrenia

Jaspreet S. Brar

Introduction

This chapter reviews the epidemiology of schizophrenia spectrum and other psychotic disorders. The spectrum includes schizophrenia, schizotypal personality disorder, delusional disorder, brief psychotic disorder, schizophreniform disorder, schizoaffective disorder, substance/medication-induced psychotic disorder, psychotic disorder due to another medical condition, catatonia, and other (specified and unspecified) schizophrenia spectrum and other psychotic disorder (American Psychiatric Association, 2013). Schizophrenia, the commonest disorder in the spectrum, is the focus of this review. Differences between spectrum disorders, where present, are highlighted.

Incidence and Prevalence

Table 3.1 summarizes common epidemiological measures of disease frequency and burden.

Estimates of incidence and prevalence define the distribution of a disease and its determinants. Clinicians, epidemiologists,

Table 3.1 Definition of Epidemiological Terms

Measure	Definition
Incidence	A measure of new cases of disease in a population at risk in a specified period of time.
Prevalence	A measure of all cases of disease, new and existing, in a population at risk in a specified period of time. Point prevalence is an estimate of the number of new cases at any given point in time.
Effect Size	A measure of the strength of association between risk factor (exposure) and disease (outcome). It is based on comparison of the incidence of disease in a population with exposure to risk factor (at risk) to the incidence of disease in a population without exposure (not at risk).
Odds Ratio	An effect size comparing the odds of disease (outcome) given a particular risk factor (exposure) to the odds of disease in the absence of that risk factor. It is calculated for retrospective, case-control studies. Odds ratios can establish only association, not causation.
Relative Risk	An effect size comparing the risk of disease (outcome) given a particular risk factor (exposure) to the risk of disease in the absence of the risk factor. It is calculated for prospective, cohort studies. A relative risk may be used for establishing causality.
Population Attributable Risk	Also known as "population attributable fraction"; it is the number or proportion of cases of disease that would not occur if there was no exposure to the risk factor.

policy makers, and insurers use this information to optimize the management of, and reduce disease burden through, prevention and appropriate allocation of resources.

A World Health Organization (WHO) study of 10 countries estimated the annual incidence rate of schizophrenia to be between the ranges of 0.1–0.4 per 1,000 population (Jablensky et al., 1992). The lifetime prevalence of schizophrenia is estimated to be between the ranges of 0.3–0.7% (McGarth, 2008). The prevalence of schizophreniform disorder is essentially similar to that of schizophrenia, although lower rates may be observed in the United States and other developed countries (Bromet et al., 2011). About a third of cases diagnosed with schizophreniform disorder may recover completely, whereas two-thirds may progress to a diagnosis of schizophrenia. The lifetime prevalence of schizoaffective disorder is estimated to be 0.3%, with higher rates in females than in males (Perälä et al., 2007). Nine percent of cases with first episode of psychosis meet criteria for brief psychotic disorder (Susser et al., 1995). Brief psychotic disorder, also known as "brief reactive psychosis," is diagnosed if there is complete resolution of symptoms within one month of onset. If symptoms persist beyond one month, other diagnoses (for example, schizophreniform disorder or schizophrenia) are considered. Seven percent to 25% of cases with first episode of psychosis meet criteria for substance/medication-induced psychotic disorder (Crebbin et al., 2009). The lifetime prevalence of schizotypal personality disorder is approximately 3.9%, with higher rates in males (4.2%) than females (3.7%; Pulay et al., 2009).

The incidence and prevalence rates of schizophrenia have been estimated using a variety of methods. These include chart reviews and evaluation of patients in hospitals and clinics or of those receiving outpatient services. The rates estimated by these methods are based upon individuals who are receiving services. Therefore, these rates may be an underestimation.

Factors Affecting Incidence and Prevalence

Differences in incidence rates may result from differences in case-definition and case-finding methodologies. The use of different diagnostic criteria and definitions of adulthood may produce different estimates. Furthermore, diagnostic formulations based on interviews may have both a reporting and a recall bias (Takayanagi et al., 2014). Variations in prevalence rates are often a result of differences in recovery, migration rates, and mortality rates in individuals with schizophrenia.

Males usually develop the illness in their middle twenties, whereas females develop it in their late twenties (McGarth et al., 2008). The average age of onset of disease is between 20 and 25 years for males and between 25 and 30 years for females. Individuals with a family history of schizophrenia and those with a history of obstetrical complications during birth may have an earlier age of onset.

Several studies have shown geographical variations in the rates of schizophrenia. The rates of schizophrenia are higher in industrialized countries than in underdeveloped countries. Studies have also shown that individuals with schizophrenia have a more favorable course and outcome in under-developed than in industrialized countries (Leff et al., 1992). It has been argued, however, that these findings may result from an association between increased mortality among those in underdeveloped countries who have a poorer prognosis.

A systematic review of 55 studies examining the incidence of schizophrenia shows that rates of the disease are higher among males than females, with a median male/female rate ratio of 1.4 (McGrath et al., 2004). Only nine of the studies included in this review showed higher rates in females versus males. Gender differences in the rates of schizophrenia may be confounded by a higher propensity for males to get hospitalized (Munk-Jørgensen, 1985).

The incidence of schizophrenia is also higher among migrants compared to the native-born (McGarth et al., 2014). The median migrant/native-born rate ratio is 4.6.

The rates of schizophrenia are also higher among some geographical regions and groups. While higher prevalence rates have been observed in northern Finland, Sweden, and parts of Ireland, lower rates have been found among the Amish and Hutterites in North America (1.2 per 1,000 population; Nimgaonkar et al., 2000).

Risk Factors

Several factors can modify the risk for developing the disease. These can generally be classified into risk indicators, proxy variables, and putative risk factors. The risk indicators are factors that precede the development of disease but are not causally related to it. Proxy variables are factors that are related to another risk-modifying factor and precede the development of disease but are not causally related to it. Putative risk factors are generally considered to be causally related to the development of disease.

The risk indicators include delayed developmental milestones and cognitive, behavioral, and social deficits that manifest in early or later childhood. In addition, structural brain abnormalities such as enlarged ventricles and diminished amygdala-hippocampus volume also increase the risk for development of the disease. Soft neurological signs and minor physical and dermatoglyphic anomalies are also associated with the risk of developing schizophrenia. This chapter reviews proxy variables and putative risk factors associated with the development of schizophrenia. A summary of risk factors is presented in Table 3.2.

Table 3.2 Risk Factors for Schizophrenia

1. Sociodemographic Factors	2. Developmental Factors
a. Gender	a. Perinatal factors:
b. Paternal age	i. Infections
c. Marital status	ii. Nutrition
d. Social class	iii. Maternal stress
e. Migrant status	iv. Obstetric complications
f. Urbanicity	v. Season of birth
g. Ethnicity and race	b. Experiences during childhood and adolescence
	c. Alcohol and recreational drugs
	d. Genetics

Sociodemographic Factors

Gender

Some, but not all, studies have shown that females have a milder form of the disease than males do. Males are also more likely to have negative symptoms than females are (Roy et al., 2001). Several mechanisms have been proposed to explain gender differences, mainly focusing on the modulatory effect of estrogen on dopamine receptors and the faster pace of brain maturation in females prior to the development of the disease. These factors may also explain why the age of onset of disease in females is later than in males. The favorable course in females may result from a later onset of the disease, which may in turn have resulted from better premorbid functioning and social supports. Females, however, have higher incidence rates of schizoaffective disorder than males, which is consistent with higher rates of depression among females (Malhi et al., 2008).

Paternal Age

A strong association between the advancing age of the father and the development of schizophrenia in the offspring has been observed (Reichenberg et al, et al., 2002). It has been proposed that the risk in offspring of older fathers may result from de novo mutations (Malaspina et al., 2001).

Marital Status

The risk of developing schizophrenia is higher among unmarried individuals than among those who are married. Several possible reasons have been suggested. Unmarried individuals, especially males, who have an earlier age of onset and have poor premorbid functioning may self-select against marriage. Furthermore, the close support provided through marriage may shield at-risk individuals from developing the disease.

Social Class

Lower social class is associated with a higher risk of developing schizophrenia, especially in industrialized countries. This may be a function of the poor quality of maternal and obstetrical care, higher likelihood of exposure to infectious agents, high stress, and other factors related to impoverished environments. On the other hand, vulnerable individuals or those who have recently developed schizophrenia may show a gradual downward drift in their social class. This phenomenon is often referred to as "the selection–drift hypothesis." Vulnerable individuals are thus prevented from achieving higher social class. It remains unclear whether social factors are a risk or an epiphenomenon that results from having the disease.

Migrant Status

Migrant status is a proxy variable associated with the disease. Migration, especially in the first generation of immigrants, increases the risk for schizophrenia. Possible reasons include psychosocial stress antecedent to migration and misdiagnosis resulting from cultural and language differences. The prevalence rates tend to approximate the population means after the first generation. Subsequent generations of Afro-Caribbean immigrants to the United Kingdom, however, have shown higher rates of schizophrenia than the previous generations and prove to be an exception to this finding (Sugarman & Craufurd, 1994).

Urbanicity

Place of birth is a proxy variable associated with the disease. Individuals born and raised in urban areas are at higher risk for developing schizophrenia than those born in rural areas. Danish population-based studies report a relative risk of about 2.4 for the urban-born but a considerably larger population attributable risk of 34.6% (Mortensen et al., 1999).

Ethnicity and Race

Older studies have shown higher prevalence rates of schizophrenia among African Americans, but these have been attributable to a racially based diagnostic bias. The prevalence rate of schizophrenia among African Americans and other non-white racial groups is more recently observed to be no different from the general population's.

Developmental Risk Factors

The neurodevelopmental model hypothesizes that the disease is related to changes in normal brain development. These changes may occur in the pre- or perinatal periods.

Perinatal Factors

Maternal health conditions such as preeclampsia have been shown to increase the risk of schizophrenia (Byrne et al., 2007). Prenatal factors have been implicated in the development of schizophrenia.

a. *Infections*: Infections, especially during the second trimester, increase the risk for schizophrenia (Brown et al., 2006). The effects of various infections are presented in Table 3.3.

Table 3.3 Infections During Pregnancy and Estimated
Effect Size

Type of Infection	Estimated Effect Size
Influenza	2.0
Poliomyelitis	1.1
Respiratory infections	2.1
Rubella	5.2
Toxoplasmosis	2.6

Furthermore, childhood infections involving the central
nervous system during infancy can also increase the risk for
schizophrenia (Koponen et al., 2004).

b. *Nutrition*: Suboptimal nutrition, especially in the first and
second trimester, can increase the risk for schizophrenia
in offspring. Among possible causes are low maternal
folate, low prenatal vitamin D, and deficits in specific
micronutrients. A two-fold higher risk of schizophrenia
was observed in the offspring of women who were
pregnant during the 1944–1945 famine in Holland (Susser &
Lin, 1992).

c. *Maternal stress*: Exposure to stressful life events such
as bereavement, war, floods, etc., increases the risk for
schizophrenia. This is probably mediated by maternal
cortisol, an excess of which may have toxic effects on the
hippocampus of the fetus. The effects of various stressors
are presented in Table 3.4.

Table 3.4 Maternal Stress and Estimated Effect Size

Maternal Stress	Estimated Effect Size
Death of a spouse	6.2
Floods	1.8
Unwanted pregnancy	2.4
Depression	1.8

d. *Obstetrical complications*: Hypoxia, low birth weight, and preterm birth increase the risk of developing schizophrenia. The risk may further increase if there are complications during labor and delivery. The evidence for obstetrical complications, however, is inconclusive because of methodological problems related to measurement issues; mainly recall biases. Low birth weight and preterm birth may result from problems with intrauterine growth that may disrupt normal brain development.

e. *Season of birth*: Season of birth is a proxy variable associated with the disease. Individuals born during winter or early spring months are at increased risk for schizophrenia. There may be higher maternal exposure to winter-borne viruses, and births at this time of the year are more likely to be exposed to winter infections. Furthermore, in the Northern Hemisphere, lower levels of winter sunlight may be an additional contributor to the increased risk. The Danish linkage study has shown that a small excess of births in the winter (relative risk = 1.1) may yield a large population attributable risk (10.5%; Mortensen et al., 1999).

Experiences During Childhood and Adolescence

Severe psychosocial stressors such as loss of a parent, social isolation, traumatic brain injury, or other forms of trauma including physical and sexual and neglect, are associated with a higher risk for developing schizophrenia. Childhood infections involving the central nervous system can increase the risk for schizophrenia fourfold.

Alcohol and Recreational Drugs

The use of alcohol and recreational drugs, mainly cannabis, cocaine, and amphetamines, can also increase the risk for schizophrenia. Although the evidence for dopamine-releasing agents like cocaine and amphetamines' leading to increased risk is equivocal, there is substantial support for the association between cannabis use and the rapid precipitation and onset of disease in genetically vulnerable individuals. The working hypothesis for this association postulates that the endocannabinoid system, which is responsible for neurodevelopment and neuroplasticity, is interfered with by tetrahydrocannabinol (THC) in exogenously consumed cannabis. Furthermore, the dose–response relationship is supported by the observation that early onset of cannabis use affords a higher risk of developing the disease. Longitudinal studies, however, are required to conclusively establish the association and quantify the magnitude of risk.

Table 3.5 Relative Risk of Schizophrenia Among Relatives of Individuals with Schizophrenia

First-degree Relatives	Second-degree Relatives
Monozygotic twins 48%	Half-sibling 6%
Dizygotic twins 17%	Grandchildren 5%
Children 13%	Nephews and nieces 4%
Siblings 9%	Aunts and uncles 2%
Two parents 27%	First cousin 2%
One parent 7%	Grandparent 4%

Genetic Factors

The majority of individuals with schizophrenia do not have a family history of the illness. However, the rates of disease are higher among those who have first- and second-degree relatives with schizophrenia. The risk varies depending upon how closely related the individual is to the affected relative. In monozygotic twins whose genetic constitution is identical, only moderately high concordance rates of schizophrenia in both twins have been observed. If one monozygotic twin is affected with schizophrenia, the relative risk for the other twin to develop the disease is about 48%. Furthermore, the relative risk associated with having two parents with schizophrenia is about 46%. This suggests that non-genetic environmental factors play an important role in the development of schizophrenia. The relative risks associated with other first- and second-degree relatives are presented in Table 3.5 (Gottesman, 1991).

It is known that the transmission of schizophrenia is mediated by genes rather than by adoptive relationships. Many genes may be implicated in its transmission rather than any single gene. Genetic factors may determine an individual's susceptibility, but environmental factors may determine whether or not the disease manifests. The diathesis–stress model for causation has been proposed to explain how genetic and other factors collectively increase the risk for schizophrenia (Neuchterlein & Dawson, 1986). According to this model, the disease develops when a threshold of vulnerability determined by genetic factors and other factors (e.g., psychosocial stress) is exceeded.

Protective Factors

An inverse correlation between rheumatoid arthritis and schizophrenia has been observed in several studies, leading to the speculation that these two disorders develop through common immune pathways such that the development of one disorder confers protection (immunity) against the development of the other (Torrey & Yolken, 2001). A decreased incidence of schizophrenia has also been observed among individuals with type-1 diabetes (Juvonen et al., 2007). A similar association with other autoimmune diseases has not been demonstrated. A protective effect of diet containing omega-3 fatty acids during the pre- and postnatal periods to prevent the development of schizophrenia has been proposed but not empirically tested.

Psychiatric and Physical Comorbidities in Schizophrenia

Psychiatric Comorbidities

Depression, substance abuse, and anxiety frequently co-occur with schizophrenia (Buckley et al., 2009; Cosoff & Hafner, 1998). Rates for common comorbid conditions are presented in Table 3.6.

The rates of comorbid psychiatric conditions may be underestimated in cases experiencing first-episode psychosis due to the hierarchy in diagnostic formulation, where a diagnosis of schizophrenia may supplant one of depression and anxiety.

Suicidal ideation and behavior occur frequently in schizophrenia, with higher rates among young males, especially for those with comorbid substance abuse. It is estimated that 20% of patients with schizophrenia may have made at least one suicide attempt (Hawton et al., 2005). The lifetime risk for suicide in people with schizophrenia is around 5% (Hor and & Taylor, 2010). Suicidal ideation and behavior may result from command hallucinations to harm oneself, or from depression and feelings of hopelessness.

Individuals with schizophrenia are more likely to be victims rather than perpetrators of homicide, and the overall amount of violence—including homicide—that can be attributed to individuals with schizophrenia remains very small. Recent research,

Table 3.6 Rates of Comorbid Psychiatric Disorders

Comorbid Disorder	Rate
Depressive disorder	50%
Substance abuse	47%
Panic disorder	15%
Post-traumatic stress disorder	29%
Obsessive-compulsive disorder	23%
Generalized anxiety disorder	12%
Any anxiety disorder	43%

however, suggests that individuals with schizophrenia may have an increased risk of committing violent acts, including homicide. A recent systematic review found that the risk of homicide (as perpetrators) in persons with schizophrenia was 0.3% compared with 0.02% in the general population (Fazel et al., 2009). Much, although not all, of the excess risk may be attributable to comorbid substance abuse. Other risk factors include young age, male gender, low socioeconomic status, a history of violence, recent stressful life event, severity of symptoms, and poor adherence to medications.

Physical Comorbidities

A clustering of factors leading to poor health outcomes is common in schizophrenia. The prevalence of smoking is two- to four-fold higher among patients with schizophrenia than among the general population, with smoking rates approaching 80% (Hughes et al., 2000). Obesity resulting from poor nutrition, psychotropic medications, and sedentary lifestyles is observed at rates four times higher than in the general population (Vancampfort et al., 2013). Furthermore, the propensity of several second-generation antipsychotics to cause weight gain and glucose dysregulation has increased the rates of obesity-related medical comorbidities in the last two decades. Together with the high rates of smoking, the rates of common cardiovascular diseases are considerably higher in schizophrenia (Table 3.7).

The rates of viral diseases, including hepatitis; respiratory diseases, including tuberculosis, pneumonia, and chronic obstructive pulmonary disease; some cancers; musculoskeletal diseases,

Table 3.7 Risk of Comorbid Physical Disorders Compared to General Population

Comorbid Disorder	Odds Ratio
Hypertension	1.4
Low high-density lipoprotein (HDL)	2.4
Hypertriglyceridemia	2.7
Metabolic syndrome	2.4
Diabetes	2.0

including osteoporosis; oral diseases related to poor dental health; and poor pregnancy outcomes are higher in schizophrenics than in the general population (DeHert et al., 2011). Outcomes related to medical illnesses are made worse due to inadequate involvement in primary, secondary, and tertiary physical health care.

Mortality in Schizophrenia

There is convergent evidence that individuals with schizophrenia have a two-fold to three-fold higher mortality compared with the general population. This excess mortality corresponds to a 10–25-year reduction in life expectancy. Studies examining mortality in schizophrenia have shown that physical illnesses—mainly cardiovascular diseases that result from modifiable lifestyle risk factors, including poor diet and nutrition, smoking, alcohol, and substance use and sedentary living—exert a greater influence on mortality than the risk associated with suicide or the adverse effects of antipsychotic medications (Laursen et al., 2012; Laursen, 2011).

Conclusion

The epidemiological risk and prognostic factors associated with schizophrenia overlap with those of other spectrum disorders; namely, schizotypal personality disorder, delusional disorder, brief psychotic disorder, schizophreniform disorder, schizoaffective disorder, substance/medication-induced psychotic disorder, psychotic disorder due to another medical condition, and catatonia associated with another mental disorder. Differences, where present, have been highlighted in the chapter. These disorders may differ from one another with respect to onset, phenomenology, duration of symptoms, and degree of psychopathology, but several disorders, such as schizoaffective disorder, are not distinct nosological categories. At present, the epidemiology of schizophrenia focuses on studying risk and prognostic factors associated with newer antipsychotic agents with the intention of minimizing treatment-related medical comorbidities and improving the quality of life for individuals with schizophrenia.

Self-Learning Questions

1. Onset of psychotic symptoms in schizophrenia is:
   a. Earlier in males
   b. Often triggered by stressful life events
   c. Often preceded by non-psychotic prodromal symptoms for weeks or months
   d. Usually during adolescence or early adulthood
   e. All of the above

2. All of the following increase a person's risk for developing schizrenia, EXCEPT:
   a. Being female
   b. Having a twin with schizophrenia
   c. Being born in a city
   d. Being born in the winter
   e. Using cannabis heavily as a teen

3. Which of the following statements most accurately describes the way schizophrenia appears to be transmitted through families?
   a. First- and second-generation relatives increase relative risk by about the same amount.
   b. Genetic factors appear to carry the greatest influence in transmission of the illness, with very little role for environmental factors.
   c. Having a monozygotic twin with the illness increases risk more than having a dizygotic twin with the illness.
   d. Having an aunt or uncle with schizophrenia does not increase a person's risk for developing the illness beyond the base rate in the population as a whole.

4. When discussing smoking with a patient with a psychotic disorder, which statement would be most accurate?
   a. Although smoking rates may be higher, the increase in general medical comorbidity appears to have little relationship to tobacco use.
   b. Individuals with psychotic disorders smoke at about the same rate as the general population.
   c. Smoking rates are higher in this group compared to the general population, about 35%.
   d. Upwards of 80% of patients with psychotic disorders smoke.

Key Learning Points

- Lifetime prevalence of psychotic disorders ranges from 0.3% for schizoaffective disorder to 3.9% for schizotypal personality disorder, with schizophrenia being 0.5%. For schizophrenia, males are at slightly higher risk and tend to have a slightly earlier onset, in their early twenties.
- There are numerous risk factors for the development of schizophrenia, both *sociodemographic* (lower socioeconomic status, urbanicity, migrant status, etc.) and *developmental* (perinatal infection/stress, obstetrical complications, family history, cannabis use, traumatic life events, etc.).
- Comorbidity is common in individuals with psychotic disorders, particularly depression, anxiety, addiction, and a variety of physical health conditions (especially metabolic, cardiovascular, and viral).

108 **Schizophrenia and Related Disorders**

References

American Psychiatric Association. (2013). *The Diagnostic and Statistical Manual of Mental Disorders: DSM-5*, Washington, D.C: American Psychiatric Association.

Bromet, E. J., Kotov, R., Fochtmann, L. J., Carlson, G. A., Tanenberg-Karant, M., Ruggero, C., & Chang, S. W. (2011). Diagnostic shifts during the decade following first admission for psychosis. *American Journal of Psychiatry, 168*, 1186–1194.

Brown, A. S. (2006). Prenatal infection as a risk factor for schizophrenia. *Schizophrenia Bulletin, 32*(2), 200–202.

Buckley, P. F., Miller, B. J., Lehrer, D. S., & Castle, D. J. (2009). Psychiatric comorbidities and schizophrenia. *Schizophrenia Bulletin, 35*(2), 383–402.

Byrne, M., Agerbo, E., Bennedsen, B., Eaton, W. W., & Mortensen, P. B. (2007). Obstetric conditions and risk of first admission with schizophrenia: A Danish National Register based study. *Schizophrenia Research, 97*(1), 51–59.

Cosoff, S. J., & Julian Hafner, R. (1998). The prevalence of comorbid anxiety in schizophrenia, schizoaffective disorder and bipolar disorder. *Australian and New Zealand Journal of Psychiatry, 32*(1), 67–72.

Crebbin, K., Mitford, E., Paxton, R., & Turkington, D. (2009). First-episode drug-induced psychosis: A medium term follow up study reveals a high-risk group. *Social Psychiatry and Psychiatric Epidemiology, 44*(9), 710–715.

De Hert, M., Vancampfort, D., Correll, C. U., Mercken, V., Peuskens, J., Sweers, K., & Mitchell, A. J. (2011). Guidelines for screening and monitoring of cardiometabolic risk in schizophrenia: Systematic evaluation. *The British Journal of Psychiatry, 199*(2), 99–105.

Fazel, S., Gulati, G., Linsell, L., Geddes, J. R., & Grann, M. (2009). Schizophrenia and violence: Systematic review and meta-analysis. *PLoS Medicine, 6*(8), 929.

Gottesman, I. I. (1991). *Schizophrenia Genesis: The Origin of Madness*. New York: Freeman.

Hawton, K., Sutton, L., Haw, C., Sinclair, J., & Deeks, J. J. (2005). Schizophrenia and suicide: Systematic review of risk factors. *The British Journal of Psychiatry, 187*(1), 9–20.

Hor, K., & Taylor, M. (2010). Suicide and schizophrenia: A systematic review of rates and risk factors. *Journal of Psychopharmacology, 24*(4), 81–90.

Jablensky, A., Sartorius, N., Ernberg, G., Anker, M., Korten, A., Cooper, J. E., & Bertelsen, A. (1992). Schizophrenia: Manifestations, incidence, and course in different cultures. A World Health Organization Ten-Country Study. *Psychological Medicine. Monograph Supplement, 20*, 1–97.

Juvonen, H., Reunanen, A., Haukka, J., Muhonen, M., Suvisaari, J., Arajärvi, R., & Lönnqvist, J. (2007). Incidence of schizophrenia in a nationwide cohort of patients with type 1 diabetes mellitus. *Archives of General Psychiatry, 64*(8), 894–899.

Koponen, H., Veijola, J., Jones, P., Jokelainen, J., & Isohanni, M. (2004). Childhood central nervous system infections and risk for schizophrenia. *European Archives of Psychiatry and Clinical Neuroscience, 254*(1), 9–13.

Laursen, T. M. (2011). Life expectancy among persons with schizophrenia or bipolar affective disorder. *Schizophrenia Research, 131*(1), 101–104.

Laursen, T. M., Munk-Olsen, T., & Vestergaard, M. (2012). Life expectancy and cardiovascular mortality in persons with schizophrenia. *Current Opinion in Psychiatry, 25*(2), 83–88.

Leff, J., Sartorius, N., Jablensky, A., Korten, A., & Ernberg, G. (1992). The International Pilot Study of Schizophrenia: Five-year follow-up findings. *Psychological Medicine, 22*(01), 131–145.

Malaspina, D., Harlap, S., Fennig, S., Heiman, D., Nahon, D., Feldman, D., & Susser, E. S. (2001). Advancing paternal age and the risk of schizophrenia. *Archives of General Psychiatry*, *58*(4), 361–367.

Malhi, G. S., Green, M., Fagiolini, A., Peselow, E. D., & Kumari, V. (2008). Schizoaffective disorder: Diagnostic issues and future recommendations. *Bipolar Disorders*, *10*(1p2), 215–230.

McGrath, J. J., Petersen, L., Agerbo, E., Mors, O., Mortensen, P. B., & Pedersen, C. B. (2014). A comprehensive assessment of parental age and psychiatric disorders. *Journal of the American Medical Association Psychiatry*, *71*, 301–309.

McGrath, J. J., Saha, S., Welham, J., El Saadi, O., MacCauley, C., & Chant, D. (2004). A systematic review of the incidence of schizophrenia: The distribution of rates and the influence of sex, urbanicity, migrant status and methodology. *BMC Medicine*, *2*(1), 13.

McGrath, J., Saha, S., Chant, D., & Welham, J. (2008). Schizophrenia: A concise overview of incidence, prevalence, and mortality. *Epidemiologic Reviews*, *30*(1), 67–76.

Mortensen, P. B., Pedersen, C. B., Westergaard, T., Wohlfahrt, J., Ewald, H., Mors, O., Andersen, P. K., & Melbye, M. (1999). Effects of family history and place and season of birth on the risk of schizophrenia. *New England Journal of Medicine*, *340*(8), 603–608.

Munk-Jørgensen, P. (1985). The schizophrenia diagnosis in Denmark. *Acta Psychiatrica Scandinavica*, *72*(3), 266–273.

Neuchterlein, K. H., & Dawson, M. E. (1986). A heuristic vulnerability/stress model of schizophrenic episodes. *Schizophrenia Bulletin*, *10*, 300–312.

Nimgaonkar, V. L., Fujiwara, T. M., Dutta, M., Wood, J., Gentry, K., Maendel, S., & Eaton, J. (2000). Low prevalence of psychoses among the Hutterites, an isolated religious community. *American Journal of Psychiatry*, *157*(7), 1065–1070.

Perälä, J., Suvisaari, J., Saarni, S. I., Kuoppasalmi, K., Isometsä, E., Pirkola, S., & Lönnqvist, J. (2007). Lifetime prevalence of psychotic and bipolar I disorders in a general population. *Archives of General Psychiatry*, *64*(1), 19–28.

Pulay, A. J., Stinson, F. S., Dawson, D. A., Goldstein, R. B., Chou, S. P., Huang, B., & Grant, B. F. (2009). Prevalence, correlates, disability, and comorbidity of DSM-IV schizotypal personality disorder: Results from the wave 2 national epidemiologic survey on alcohol and related conditions. *Primary Care Companion to the Journal of Clinical Psychiatry*, *11*(2), 53.

Reichenberg, A., Weiser, M., Rabinowitz, J., Caspi, A., Schmeidler, J., Mark, M., & Davidson, M. (2002). A population-based cohort study of premorbid intellectual, language, and behavioral functioning in patients with schizophrenia, schizoaffective disorder, and nonpsychotic bipolar disorder. *American Journal of Psychiatry*, *159*(12), 2027–2035.

Roy, M. A., Maziade, M., Labbé, A., & Mérette, C. (2001). Male gender is associated with deficit schizophrenia: A meta-analysis. *Schizophrenia Research*, *47*(2), 141–147.

Sugarman, P. A., & Craufurd, D. (1994). Schizophrenia in the Afro-Caribbean community. *The British Journal of Psychiatry*, *164*(4), 474–480.

Susser, E. S., & Lin, S. P. (1992). Schizophrenia after prenatal exposure to the Dutch Hunger Winter of 1944–1945. *Archives of General Psychiatry*, *49*(12), 983–988.

Susser, E., Fennig, S., Jandorf, L., Amador, X., & Bromet, E. (1995). Epidemiology, diagnosis, and course of brief psychoses. *American Journal of Psychiatry*, *152*(12), 1743–1748.

Takayanagi, Y., Petersen, L., Laursen, T. M., Cascella, N. G., Sawa, A., Mortensen, P. B., & Eaton, W. W. (2014). Risk of schizophrenia spectrum and affective disorders associated with small for gestational age birth and height in adulthood. *Schizophrenia Research, 160*(1), 230–232.

Torrey, E. F., & Yolken, R. H. (2001). The schizophrenia–rheumatoid arthritis connection: Infectious, immune, or both? *Brain, Behavior, and Immunity, 15*(4), 401–410.

Vancampfort, D., Probst, M., Scheewe, T., De Herdt, A., Sweers, K., Knapen, J., & De Hert, M. (2013). Relationships between physical fitness, physical activity, smoking, and metabolic and mental health parameters in people with schizophrenia. *Psychiatry Research, 207*(1), 25–32.

Course, Prognosis, and Outcomes of Schizophrenia and Related Disorders

Konasale M. Prasad

Introduction

There is nothing more important to the physician, patients, and their families, after a diagnosis is made, than the course and outcome of a disorder. The impact of a diagnosis is mainly determined by the nature and the quality of the outcome, which depends, in large part, on the availability of effective treatments. Schizophrenia is no exception to this. Understanding the general course and outcome of schizophrenia is particularly critical for providers because devastating misconceptions about the disorder and its outcome can be demoralizing for patients and families and even impede effective treatment.

Schizophrenia and related psychotic disorders are often classified as severe mental illnesses. It is important to understand the degree of severity of this illness compared to other medical disorders. A recent large study with data from across the globe rated 220 disorders for non-fatal outcomes by assigning disability weights between 0 and 1, where 0 means no disability and 1 is the severest disability, equivalent to death (Salomon et al., 2012). The severest of all 220 rated disorders was acute schizophrenia (0.76), followed by severe multiple sclerosis (0.71). To provide a contrast, it can be noted that mild infection got a disability weight of 0.005, mild anemia scored 0.01, and metastasized cancer 0.48. It must be emphasized here that these numbers need to be interpreted appropriately, and the reader is urged to refer to the cited study (Salomon et al., 2012). These statistics are important to remember in order to validate the difficulties patients and families face in coping with the challenges of schizophrenia and to help emphasize the importance of treatment. Providers must also take care, when disseminating information about disease morbidity to patients and families, to not diminish the sense of hope in treatment that is fundamental to mental health recovery.

To better understand schizophrenia's course, prognosis, and outcomes, we will first examine two very important conceptual issues. The first is the natural evolution of the symptoms of schizophrenia, and the second is the natural course of the disorder without any modern interventions to alter its course. Deeper understanding of the evolution of the disorder will help one grasp surprising yet unpredictable variabilities in treatment response and outcomes of schizophrenia. Knowledge of the natural evolution of the disease and various antecedents to neurodevelopmental processes provides us with insight into the neurobiological underpinnings of the disorder.

You will learn that schizophrenia is closely intertwined with brain growth and development, and we will identify potential protective factors. Understanding the natural course of the disorder is important to demystify the myths of therapeutic nihilism associated with the diagnosis and its consequent social stigma. Such knowledge further prepares the astute clinician for the natural ups and downs of the disease, factors associated with such variations in the disease course, the relapses and the remissions, so as to better tailor treatment to individual patients.

Natural Evolution of Schizophrenia

There is a fairly wide consensus that schizophrenia is related to altered development of the brain, which in turn suggests that schizophrenia is likely to be a neurodevelopmental disorder. The pathology underlying schizophrenia starts well before a clinical diagnosis can even be suspected. By the time the disease clinically manifests and a patient is brought to medical attention, the pathology and the pathophysiological processes that started several years earlier are in full swing (Figure 4.1). However, the precise timing of the beginnings of the pathology, probably in response to etiological factors affecting neurodevelopment, is highly debated. The etiological factors in question could either be acting early in the neurodevelopment—even prenatally and/ or during the early postnatal period, (Modestin, Huber, Satirli, Malti, & Hell, 2003; Warner, 2004) or later, during adolescence (Feinberg, 1982). These models are aptly and respectively termed the "early hit" model and the "late hit" model. While there is evidence to support both models, observable changes in neurocognitive, behavioral, and functional domains, notwithstanding findings from postmortem neuropathology, neuroimaging, and electrophysiological studies, all converge to support the early hit model (Murray & Lewis, 1987; Weinberger, 1987). That

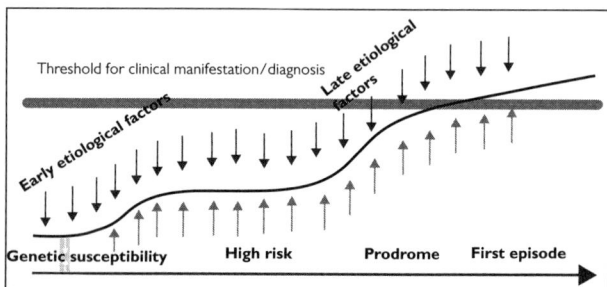

Figure 4.1 *Evolution of schizophrenia pathophysiology over the years*: Although the clinical onset is delayed until adolescence or adulthood, the pathophysiological events may be active and the neural pathways are likely to be "well established" much before the clinical manifestation.

suggests that neural pathways are well "established" by the time the illness manifests.

While the neurobiological underpinnings of schizophrenia are under active study, much more is known about the "exophenotypical" characteristics—overt manifestations of illness—that are of interest to a keen clinician. Neurobiology has begun to better inform this body of knowledge. Emerging evidence over the last four decades has confirmed clinical findings and strongly suggests that cognitive impairments are the core deficits in schizophrenia. Children, adolescents, and young adults who go on to develop schizophrenia have been repeatedly shown to perform well below age-matched comparison subjects on several standardized intelligence measures. Impairments in specific cognitive domains of attention, certain forms of memory, and decision-making abilities called "executive function" have also been reported, suggesting that these deficits are not just generalized impairments in cognitive processing, but affect certain domains more severely than others. Such deficits—both in intelligence and in specific cognitive domains—are present before the illness onset and are observed during both acute periods of the illness and in remissions. However, it is not clear whether the cognitive deficits remain stable throughout the illness or show some degree of deterioration during the illness; early evidence appears to suggest the latter, further emphasizing the need for early detection of schizophrenia and treatment; especially because of the adverse impact of cognitive deficits on long-term outcomes. Cognitive deficits more robustly predict the long-term outcome of schizophrenia than either the positive or the negative symptoms of the disorder. In fact, deficits in specific domains such as verbal memory and executive function, along with some others, may even contribute up to 60% of the variance for poor outcome.

Understanding the natural evolution of the disease is critical for another clinically relevant reason. The majority of the studies on the duration of the illness have shown it to be another important predictor of outcome for schizophrenia (Penttila, Jaaskelainen, Hirvonen, Isohanni, & Miettunen, 2014; Wyatt, 1995). The longer the duration of the illness, particularly untreated illness, the poorer the outcome. This further emphasizes the importance of early detection and treatment. However, the challenge is in the early detection. How early in life can we detect schizophrenia? Are there reliable signs and symptoms for early detection of schizophrenia? What are the sensitivity and specificity of these criteria?

A set of behavioral symptoms that may predate the onset of schizophrenia by several years has long been known, with publications on these symptoms appearing as early as 1927 (Sullivan, 1994). These early clinical manifestations of schizophrenia are often staged as *premorbid, prodromal,* and *pre-psychotic,* starting from the very early stages of the illness and extending to a behavioral state that could exist right before the full-blown expression of schizophrenia. Some of these symptoms are operationalized, and certain criteria have been proposed to more reliably identify them for research purposes. Several such criteria are published in the literature (e.g., Miller et al., 2003; Keshavan et al., 2011; Yung & McGorry, 1996). The seminal importance of identifying these behaviors is to promote early detection, which may both reduce the duration of illness, as noted, and mitigate the impact of the illness on social functioning. Even the presence of prodromal symptoms is known to reduce social functioning, and premorbid functioning itself is another known predictor of the long-term outcome of schizophrenia. Accurately determining the onset of psychosis, let alone correctly identifying a psychotic prodrome, is challenging, even with operationalized criteria for research. As such, this makes the determination of the precise duration of illness and treatment of prodromal illness very difficult. Therefore, most studies have defined the onset of illness to be the first appearance of psychotic symptoms. Even determining this can pose a challenge, though, as the determination of first appearance of psychotic symptoms requires a highly skilled interview along with plenty of collateral information.

Major Points
- Pathophysiological events are active much before the clinical manifestation of schizophrenia and may even date back to prenatal brain growth.
- Neural pathways may be "well established" by the time the treatment is initiated.
- Subtle but measurable behaviors exist years before the onset of schizophrenia in many cases; these behavioral indicators include cognitive performance as well as social adjustment and functioning.
- The importance of identifying these behaviors is underscored by their contribution to duration of illness and premorbid functioning, with both of these factors being important predictors of outcome.

Natural Course of Schizophrenia

Reported observations of different types of course and outcome in schizophrenia depend on various factors, including the definition of the disorder, diagnostic ascertainment, reliability of the diagnosis (both among diagnosticians, and by the same diagnostician over time, called *interrater* and *intrarater reliabilities*, respectively), diagnostic heterogeneity, duration of follow-up, definition of various types of recoveries and outcomes, and the interventions used.

The natural course of schizophrenia, unaffected by effective treatment interventions, was documented extensively in the pre-neuroleptic and pre–convulsive therapy era. We will discuss these findings in detail in the following subsections. Here, we must caution that the observations of this natural history depend a great deal on the definition of schizophrenia used during the time period and which world region was involved in the study. In general, American and Swiss psychiatrists, utilizing the relatively broad definition of schizophrenia originating with Eugen Bleuler, diagnosed schizophrenia five to nine times more frequently than did their British and German counterparts, using more retrospective, Kraepelinian criteria. This Kraepelinian definition of schizophrenia, which he called *dementia praecox,* emphasized cognitive decline, and was much narrower in scope. This narrower definition assumed that there may be a "nucleus" of symptoms at the core of schizophrenia driving the outcome. When considering the outcomes reported by studies, it is important to pay attention to the definition of schizophrenia used in a given study.

Although such concerns about the definition of schizophrenia are largely mitigated by the advent of official classificatory systems of diagnosis, such as the *International Classification of Diseases* (ICD) by the World Health Organization and the *Diagnostic and Statistical Manual of Mental Disorders* (DSM) by the American Psychiatric Association, the definitional issues are not completely resolved and are still a cause for concern. For example, the ICD-9, which was in use until 1992, used a broader and descriptive approach to diagnosis, as opposed to the ICD-10, which is based on a set of semi-operationalized criteria. Similarly, the DSM-I and DSM-II used more descriptive and broader definitions based on certain psychological theories compared to DSM-III and later versions, which were criteria-based and atheoretical. DSM-IV and ICD-10 also differ in their definition of psychotic disorders; whereas DSM-III and later versions use a narrower, neo-Kraepelinian concept of schizophrenia that requires at least six months of illness, ICD-10 requires only one month of illness. Thus, definitional issues are continuing to affect reliable prognostication of schizophrenia. This problem also emphasizes the need to develop more objective markers to dissect the syndrome into biologically meaningful sub-syndromes.

At this stage, the reader must be wondering how "outcome" can best be defined. As could be expected, just like with diagnosis itself, outcome has been defined differently by different groups of investigators. Mere symptom resolution for a short duration was considered by some, whereas others defined outcome based on *functional* recovery along with symptomatic improvement, and for longer durations. "Functional recovery" has generally included living independently; gainful employment with a reasonable degree of financial independence; stable housing; and having meaningful relationships, including sustaining a network of friends and relatives and being in a romantic relationship. Such conservative definitions of factors related to outcomes result in a smaller proportion of people with schizophrenia reported as having favorable outcomes (Hegarty, Baldessarini, Tohen, Waternaux, & Oepen, 1994). For example, these studies may use a complete absence of symptoms and full functional recovery for more than a few years as a definition of "full remission."

A consensus definition of "remission" in schizophrenia was proposed by a U.S. work group in 2005 (Andreasen et al., 2005). Their definition was based on using standardized research questionnaires such as the Positive and Negative Syndrome Scale (PANSS), the Brief Psychiatric Rating Scale (BPRS), the Scale for Assessment of Positive Symptoms (SAPS), and the Scale for the Assessment of Negative Symptoms (SANS). A full remission by these criteria require that the subjects score less than or equal to 2 or 3 on all items for six months or longer.

Despite frustrations at non-uniform and unstandardized definitions of improvement, recovery, and remission (e.g., Bellack, 1948), "remarkable consistencies" in outcomes have been reported in comprehensive literature reviews (e.g., Zubin et al., 1961). Older studies using narrower definitions have reported poorer outcomes ranging from 51–63%, whereas studies using broader definitions have reported better outcomes for up to 83%. The latter studies might have included several psychotic disorders that may not meet criteria for schizophrenia. In addition, the duration of follow-up also contributes to the variability in outcome data. However, newer studies that were mindful of these shortcomings have reported outcomes that could be clinically useful. In either case, it is critical to appreciate that schizophrenia is not a relentlessly progressive illness with a completely bleak long-term outcome, which should debunk therapeutic nihilism and instill hope in both the professionals and the patients.

Major Points
- For the natural course of schizophrenia, empirical data paint a rosier picture for overall outcome than does conventional belief.
- Outcome estimates depend on diagnostic ascertainment, length of follow-up, and the definition of outcome.
- Narrower diagnostic boundaries show poorer but heterogeneous outcomes.
- Longer follow-up periods provide estimates of outcome that are closer to clinical reality.
- Broad-based definition of outcome resulted in observing poorer outcomes.
- Overall, 25% of schizophrenia patients showed good to full recovery, about 50% showed moderate to considerable recovery, and another 25% continued to have residual symptoms.

Landmark Studies

Kraepelin observed in 1904 that 8–13% of dementia praecox patients had long-term full recovery, with 17% showing marked recovery. Probably owing to the narrow boundaries of "schizophrenia" as defined by Kraepelin (as discussed), and emphasizing cognitive findings, overall favorable outcome was less than 40%. This further suggest that, not only might there be a "nucleus" of symptoms driving the outcomes of schizophrenia, but cognitive deficits, particularly if progressive, may be at the core of the illness.

Length of study may also impact the outcomes. Longer-term follow-up studies report less favorable outcomes than short-term follow-ups do. A long-term follow-up study from Switzerland by Manfred Bleuler noted that 22% of patients showed full recovery using very stringent criteria, defined as near-full resolution of symptoms, full employment, and resuming social roles for five years or more. Another 51% showed moderate recovery and were less impaired but could not be considered "recovered." The rest (21%) were not able to care for themselves and were considered incapacitated. Another

4% had an atypical course that did not fit the eight different outcomes defined by Bleuler. It should be kept in mind that all of the subjects in question were diagnosed using Bleuler's broad diagnostic criteria.

In 2003, a group of Swiss investigators applied the modern diagnostic criteria (DSM-III, DSM-III-R, and DSM-IV; ICD-10 and others) to detailed chart recordings by Bleuler and found that 30% of these subjects did not meet modern criteria for schizophrenia; of these 30%, 67% met criteria for *schizoaffective disorder*. These investigators separately analyzed the schizoaffective disorder group and reanalyzed the group of people who met modern definitions of schizophrenia. This application of modern diagnostic criteria resulted in observing poorer outcomes in this group (Modestin, Huber, Satirli, Malti, & Hell, 2003). Here, 12–15% were considered recovered (similar to Kraepelin's findings), 56% were moderately recovered, and 28% were incapacitated.

An early American study from Delaware in 1955 reported similar observations in a study of institutionalized patients. After a 13-year follow-up between 1920 and 1933 of patients with schizophrenia, 24% were out of the state hospital, 65% were still in the hospital, and 11% were deceased. Interestingly, the same research group followed up another sample from 1940 to 1953, in which the subjects received the then-available treatments, including psychosurgery, convulsive treatments (ECT, Metrazol-induced seizures, and insulin coma therapy), and combinations of these treatments. They noted that about 55% of those followed were able to be discharged from the state hospital (Freyhan, 1955). No further characterization of outcome was reported.

The Vermont follow-up study is a 32-year prospective study of about 260 patients with schizophrenia that also reported about 50–66% of patients showing "full" recovery or considerable improvement at the end of the 32 years of follow-up (Harding, Brooks, Ashikaga, Strauss, & Breier, 1987a, 1987b). Interestingly, these authors compared the outcome of patients diagnosed with DSM-I, DSM-II, and DSM-III criteria and found slightly poorer outcome with DSM-III than with the broader, DSM-I–diagnosed schizophrenia.

More than a dozen studies from across the world have followed several hundred patients with schizophrenia from their first episode, for two decades or longer. These studies have remarkably observed more favorable outcomes for similar proportions of subjects, with 46–68% of patients showing "full" to "marked" recovery.

There have been multiple meta-analyses of follow-up studies, too. An excellent meta-analysis of outcomes reported in studies over the last 100 years (1895–1992), observed that about 40% of patients with schizophrenia were considered "improved" after a follow-up of about six years (Hegarty et al., 1994). Another meta-analysis of 114 studies from 1904 to 2000 that included a "recovery" criterion (complete resolution of symptoms with return to premorbid level of functioning with no restriction on the duration of recovery) concluded that 11–33% were fully recovered, while 22–53% showed only social recovery (Warner, 2004). In another meta-analysis, 40% of first-episode schizophrenia patients were noted to show recovery after a mean follow-up of about three years (Menezes, Arenovich, & Zipursky, 2006). A more recent meta-analysis that included rather stringent duration criteria for recovery reported a median proportion of recovery in just 13.5% of patients (Jaaskelainen et al., 2013). "Recovery" here was defined as a complete or nearly complete resolution of symptoms, with return to premorbid level of functioning, for a minimum of two years. Interestingly, a recent study in New York that was not part of this meta-analysis, and that followed up first-episode schizophrenia and schizoaffective disorder patients, also noted full recovery for two or more years in only 13.7%, even with modern treatments (Robinson, Woerner, McMeniman, Mendelowitz, & Bilder, 2004). Investigators here defined "full recovery" as remission from both positive and negative symptoms along with adequate social functioning that included fulfillment of age-appropriate role expectations, unsupervised performance of activities of daily living, and socially interacting. These criteria, like those of the previous meta-analysis, are more restrictive than the definition of remission proposed by the 2005 workgroup (Andreasen et al., 2005) discussed earlier in this chapter, and are very similar to Manfred Bleuler's definition of recovery. The reported low proportion of recovered patients in these studies is remarkable because of their similarity to Kraepelin's findings.

It is humbling to note that, even with advancements in the diagnosis and treatment of schizophrenia, the proportion of fully recovered patients across several studies is similar to that reported by Kraepelin more than a century ago. This suggests that the treatments for schizophrenia, including medications, may not favorably modify the pathophysiological pathways under-lying the disorder, and full restitution of neural pathways may not occur. However, it is also important to recognize that while full recovery may be uncommon, the vast majority of patients improve over time, as shown in the Vermont longitudinal study and others that follow patients out for decades. Many equate schizophrenia with Kraepelin's negative prognosis of progressive deterioration; however, actual outcomes in the literature sug-gest a more favorable prognosis, with perhaps three-quarters of patients reasonably improving over time.

Types of Outcome

Despite non-uniform definitions of *outcome* and *natural course*, certain identifiable outcome patterns have been described. There appears to be consensus on about eight different types of course and outcome described in the literature (Harding, 1988), and the DSM-5 describes seven types based on three criteria; namely, the type of onset, longitudinal course, and the end state. The end state of the illness is either full recovery, partial recov-ery, or poor recovery. For the latter two types of outcomes, in addition to poor response of psychotic symptoms (including positive and negative symptoms), functional impairments such as being unemployed, financial hardships, social isolation, and homelessness are included in determining level of recovery. Figure 4.2 illustrates five common outcomes.

As noted in a previous chapter, reduced life expectancy is a very important outcome in schizophrenia and therefore worth exploring here. Excess mortality in schizophrenia has been noted since a report in 1951 demonstrated a 3.2 times higher mortality among men and 4.8 times higher mortality among women with this disorder. These findings were based on a study that followed people with schizophrenia from 1926 to 1941 (Odegard, 1951). More recent studies have also repeatedly noted such elevated mortality rates for schizophrenia patients (Harris & Barraclough, 1998; Laursen, Nordentoft, & Mortensen, 2014). A disturb-ing trend noted in one such study (Saha, Chant, & McGrath, 2007) was that the all-causes mortality in schizophrenia was increasing in the last decade. While mortality remained high through the lifespan, another important trend was the presence of excess mortality in younger individuals, up to the age of 35. Overall, the lifespan of people with schizophrenia is shortened by 20–25 years compared to the general population's.

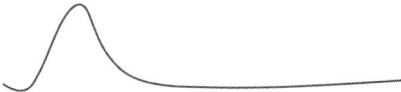

A single episode that resolves completely

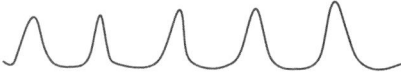

Multiple episodes that resolve almost fully with several
recurrences and relapses

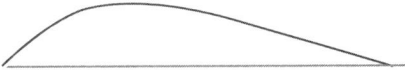

A single episode that gradually gets severe and resolves
slowly over several years

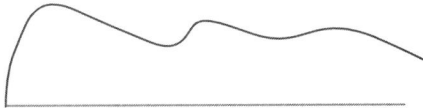

Illness that gradually gets severe and partially resolves
slowly over several years without full recovery

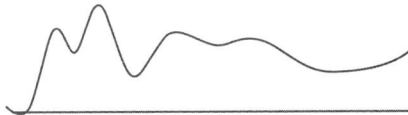

Illness with chronic undulating course with no
satisfactory remission

Figure 4.2 *Types of outcome of schizophrenia*: There are more than 5
types of outcome described in the literature. Outcomes depicted here
captures those in the literature and those specified in the DSM-5.

Four groups of factors contribute to excess mortality in
schizophrenia (Laursen et al., 2014). First among them is suicide.
It was originally thought that approximately 10% of individuals
with schizophrenia committed suicide. Large meta-analyses have

reported that 5–6% of patients with schizophrenia complete suicide (Hawton, Sutton, Haw, Sinclair, & Deeks, 2005; Palmer, Pankratz, & Bostwick, 2005), while about 20% attempt suicide (Challis, Nielssen, Harris, & Large, 2013). Another meta-analysis reported that suicides can be elevated by as high as thirteen-fold (Saha et al., 2007) (standardized mortality ratio, which is the ratio of observed deaths by suicide among schizophrenia patients to expected suicides in the general population). Clinically, it is thought that these suicides are more likely to be related to comorbid affective symptoms than to core schizophrenia features. Significant risk factors for suicide in schizophrenia are previous depressive disorder, prior suicide attempt, substance use, agitation, fear of mental disintegration, poor compliance, and recent loss. Males had a higher risk, while other sociodemographic factors such as ethnicity, marital status, and employment status were not significant (Hawton et al., 2005).

The other factors contributing to excess mortality in schizophrenia are related to physical health. First, somatic illnesses either go undetected or are detected in late stages among persons with this disorder. This contributes to the increased natural-cause mortality seen in this population. The Charlson Index, adopted from breast cancer studies, showed that 19 of the 20 somatic disorders examined showed elevated prevalence among persons with schizophrenia (Laursen, Munk-Olsen, & Gasse, 2011). In addition to underdetection of somatic illnesses, increased vulnerability to chronic medical disorders has been reported for subjects with schizophrenia (Laursen, Munk-Olsen, & Vestergaard, 2012). Second, the use of antipsychotics may be a risk factor for excess mortality. Antipsychotics have been associated with increased risk of metabolic syndrome, sudden death, and myocarditis. Some studies have not replicated these associations, however. Longer-term studies are needed to clearly establish this relationship, as well as to estimate the risk attributable to different antipsychotics. Finally, increased risk of mortality in schizophrenia is also associated with lifestyle factors, including increased frequency of smoking, insufficient physical exercise, and poor dietary habits.

The association of violence with schizophrenia and related psychotic disorders has also received enormous attention in the media and so deserves our attention here as a potential illness outcome. It was once thought that the risk for violence in persons with schizophrenia and related psychotic disorders was no more than that found in the general population. Large studies, however, questioned this notion. Current data suggest that there is a modest association between these disorders and violence (Kooyman, Dean, Harvey, & Walsh, 2007). Existing studies report wide variations in such associations, though, which muddies the picture. For example, the odds ratio (ratio of the odds of violence by patients with schizophrenia to violence by individuals who are not mentally ill) varies between 1 and 7 for men, and 4 and 29 for women (Fazel, Gulati, Linsell, Geddes, & Grann, 2009). Overall, studies suggest that the odds ratio for violence by schizophrenia patients is elevated (approximately 4 for men and 8 for women), with such associations being strongest among schizophrenia patients with substance use. Interestingly, the elevated risk among schizophrenia patients who were substance users was similar to the violence risk for substance users without psychosis (Fazel et al., 2009). The reasons for such variations include study designs, the populations examined in these studies, the definition of schizophrenia used, the definition of violence, data-collection methods (self-reports, informants, public records etc.), sociodemographic factors, and illness comorbidities.

Homicide recidivism in schizophrenia is a related issue that can be sensationalized in the media. A recent meta-analysis of three published and 11 unpublished studies reported that homicide recidivism (homicide committed after the proceedings for the previous homicide were concluded) is low (about 2.3%), less than the proportion reported in published studies (Golenkov, Nielssen, & Large, 2014). Of concern is the potential publication bias to report higher recidivism among schizophrenia patients, noted in the same meta-analysis.

Factors Contributing to the Outcome of Schizophrenia

Considering the factors discussed, prospective prediction of prognosis of schizophrenia, which is highly relevant to a clinician providing direct care, both at the time of diagnosis and during active treatment of an episode, is a complicated process. Here follows a discussion of various factors that can help prognosticate outcomes of the disorder.

Demographic Factors

Age

The earlier the age at onset, the worse the outcome. Since schizophrenia is closely intertwined with the brain development, earlier onset of the illness may suggest a more severe impairment of neurodevelopment. The basis for this proposition is supported by more severe cognitive impairments in early onset schizophrenia than is found in adult-onset illness (Frangou, 2010).

Sex

Female patients are likely to have better outcomes than male patients do. A possible explanation for this may be related to later age of onset among women. There are also suggestions that estrogen may dampen the dopamine system to some extent during the childbearing age. Since schizophrenia is considered to be related to dopamine system alterations, modulation of the dopamine system by estrogen may offer a slightly better outcome.

Socioeconomic Status

Social status by itself may not have a direct impact on outcomes. However, social status may affect outcomes through related factors such as accessibility and affordability of care, likelihood of living in a high-stress environment, and lack of understanding of the illness, among others.

Culture

There are reports of patients' having better outcomes in certain Asian cultures in which the economy is more agrarian than in industrialized countries. This association has been questioned, however. A meta-analysis recently noted that the recovery rate (defined as complete to nearly complete symptomatic recovery, along with return to premorbid levels of functioning for two or more years) in low- and/or lower-middle-income countries was, at 36.4%, nearly 3 times that observed in high and upper middle income countries, which showed 12–13% recovery rates (Jaaskelainen et al., 2013). It is possible that acceptance of illness and family support systems play a more important role within a culture than the culture itself does. More studies are needed to understand specific factors that confer better outcome in certain cultures.

Clinical Factors

Type of Onset

Patients with acute onset of illness tend to have better outcomes than do those with insidious onset. This may be related to the duration of untreated psychosis, discussed next.

Duration of Untreated Psychosis

The longer the duration of untreated illness, the poorer the outcome (Penttila et al., 2014). This is one of most replicated findings in schizophrenia research, and it bolsters the conventional medical wisdom of the importance of early diagnosis and institution of treatment. One must be careful in attempting to ascertain when the first onset of psychotic symptoms occurred. This requires considerable patience and skill at clinical interviewing, along with multiple collateral sources of information. There have been some systematic attempts to diagnostically include the onset of prodromal symptoms to mark the onset of schizophrenia (Keshavan et al., 2003). However, current evidence does not support defining the onset of illness from the appearance of prodromal symptoms to predict long-term outcome, as such efforts have not been shown to be more reliable than using the onset of psychotic symptoms for such purpose. However, this does not reduce the significance of identifying prodromal symptoms. Such characterization could play a substantial role both in the primary prevention of illness as well as in considerably shortening the duration of untreated illness. With insidious onset of illness, the patients are likely to have longer duration of illness before treatment is initiated.

Premorbid History

A well-adjusted premorbid life, before the onset of the illness, may predict better prognosis. Poor premorbid functioning may also suggest a more pernicious form of illness is present (Haas & Sweeney, 1992; Murray, O'Callaghan, Castle, & Lewis, 1992), and it has been associated with more profound cognitive deficits, more severe negative symptoms, and greater likelihood of experiencing side effects with antipsychotics (Strous et al., 2004). Premorbid functioning may also be greatly influenced by support systems, as discussed later. It is often clinically difficult to distinguish between poor premorbid functioning and the presence of prodromal symptoms. In addition, the presence of prodromal symptoms before the onset of frank illness could contribute to poorer prognosis.

Cognitive Performance

Increasingly, schizophrenia is considered a cognitive illness (Elvevag & Goldberg, 2000; Kahn & Keefe, 2013). Among the predictors of long-term social outcome, cognitive impairments are robust predictors, accounting for a substantial portion, nearly 60%, of the variance for this type of outcome. As discussed earlier, impairments in specific domains such as verbal memory and executive function are highly predictive of outcome. However, the actual variance contributed by *neurocognition* (e.g., attention, memory, perception, reasoning) ranges from 20–60% (Green, Kern, Braff, & Mintz, 2000). A significant proportion of the rest of the variance (40–80%) is associated with deficits in *social cognition* (Couture, Penn, & Roberts, 2006). Social cognition is a complex construct that is defined as a domain of cognition that involves the perception, interpretation, and processing of social information (Ostrom, 1984). Although neurocognition is required for social cognition, social cognition as a domain has been noted to be distinct from neurocognition. Unfortunately, cognitive performance is hardly assessed as part of the routine evaluation of psychotic disorders.

Family History of Psychosis

Family history of psychosis is associated both with poor premorbid functioning and with cognitive functions. In addition to the negative impact family history of psychosis can indirectly have on poor premorbid and cognitive functioning, the presence of psychosis among first-degree relatives may directly impact poorer outcomes (Jarbin, Ott, & Von Knorring, 2003; Kakela et al., 2014; Norman, Manchanda, Malla, Harricharan, & Northcott, 2007). Presence of family history of psychosis is also associated with poor response to medications (Joober et al., 2005).

Psychopathology

Using a statistical technique called *factor analysis*, schizophrenic psychopathology has been classified into three groups; namely, positive, negative, and disorganized sub-syndromes. Among these, negative symptoms are shown to be weakly predictive of long-term outcome. Interestingly, positive symptoms have the least predictive capability. The presence of depressive symptoms has been noted to predict a better prognosis. Precise reasons underlying such associations are unclear. In addition, paranoid schizophrenia is likely to be associated with better outcome than other subtypes.

Support Systems

In general, support systems can be grouped into primary, secondary, and tertiary supports. The *primary* support system refers to the immediate family; e.g., parents, siblings, partners, and children. The *secondary* support system refers to friends, colleagues, and relatives. The *tertiary* support system subsumes professional mental health services and community supports, such as peer support, interest, and focus groups, etc. The broader the support systems, and the more highly the relationships are interconnected, the better the prognosis.

Treatment-Related Factors

As mentioned earlier, the importance of early diagnosis and initiation of treatment cannot be overemphasized. Good adherence to treatment, greater tolerability of medications, and appropriate dosing all contribute to better outcomes (Figure 4.3).

Predictors of outcome in schizophrenia	
GOOD PROGNOSIS	**POOR PROGNOSIS**
• Female	• Male
• Married	• Single
• Later onset	• Early Onset
• Good premorbid history	• Poor premorbid history
• Acute onset	• Insidious onset
• Positive Symptoms	• Negative Symptoms
• Affective symptoms	• Family history of Schizophrenia
• Short duration of illness	• Long duration of illness
• Good support system	• Poor support system
• Good treatment compliance	• Poor treatment compliance
	• Cognitive Impairments

Figure 4.3 *Factors affecting course and outcome of schizophrenia*: Factors within the red box can be considered invariant factors over which physicians have minimal control, except probably for the duration of illness. Modifiable factors are outside the red box, of which cognitive impairments have the most robust evidence of contributing to poor outcome.

Given the long list of factors associated with the prognosis of schizophrenia, a precise understanding of how much weight can be assigned to each of these factors, and what combination of factors will lead to the best outcome, is nonexistent. In general, the presence of cognitive impairments, poor premorbid functioning, and poor adherence to treatment can be emphasized as more robust outcome predictors. That being said, the prediction of course and outcome of schizophrenia is not a one-time judgment but a moving target throughout the course of this chronic illness. Although a given patient may have several good prognostic indicators, early discontinuation of treatment, erratic adherence to treatment, or substance use can push the illness trajectory toward poor prognosis. Thus, prediction of prognosis is an ongoing process, just like recovery.

Other Psychotic Disorders

Brief Psychotic Disorders

Systematic studies of long-term outcome in brief psychotic disorders are lacking. Many existing studies have used their own criteria for diagnosis rather than the standard ICD or DSM definitions, making it difficult to compare across the studies. One Scandinavian study that followed brief psychotic disorder patients noted frequent diagnostic changes, making the evaluation of outcome specific to brief psychotic disorders difficult. In fact, change of diagnosis could be considered to be one of the outcomes of brief psychotic disorder. One study that followed a small number of patients with brief psychotic disorder noted significantly favorable outcomes, where about 52% of subjects were employed and 91% were living independently at the end of a mean follow-up of 7.8 years. In addition, severity of disability, psychological impairment, and overall social functioning, measured using the Global Assessment of Functioning (GAF; which is the Axis V of DSM-IV–recommended multiaxial diagnosis), were considerably more favorable for brief psychotic disorder patients compared to schizophrenia patients with positive symptoms (Pillmann, Haring, Balzuweit, & Marneros, 2002).

Delusional Disorder

To examine the impact of neuroleptics, outcomes for delusional disorder were compared between patients diagnosed during the periods extending from 1946 to 1948 and from 1958 to 1961. Investigators did not find significant differences in the outcomes between the groups, suggesting that antipsychotics may not be effective in treating delusional disorders (Opjordsmoen & Retterstol, 1993). Another follow-up study noted that more than 50% of patients with delusional disorder remained delusional at the end of eight years; they also found that many of these patients could be rediagnosed as having schizophrenia (Jorgensen, 1994). About 10% showed some improvement, and another 30% showed persistence. The onset of symptoms in delusional disorder can be acute or gradual. Only the severe forms generally come to medical attention. Delusional disorder does not lead to severe deterioration in functioning in most cases. Unlike in schizophrenia, earlier onset in delusional disorders carries a better prognosis. The rest of the prognostic factors are similar to schizophrenia's. Persecutory delusions tend to resolve better than the grandiose and jealous type of delusions.

Schizophreniform Illness

By definition, schizophreniform illness cannot continue beyond six months. However, it is important to know patient outcomes beyond six months. About 60–80% of patients diagnosed with schizophreniform illness may progress to schizophrenia. A five-year follow-up study noted 25% had fully recovered within six months, and such patients were functioning better than first-episode schizophrenia subjects. In addition, none of the patients diagnosed with schizophreniform illness required rehospitalization (Zhang-Wong, Beiser, Bean, & Iacono, 1995).

Conclusion

The course and prognosis of schizophrenia must be viewed in conjunction with the evolution of the concept of schizophrenia over the last century or more. Furthermore, the outcome of the illness needs to be understood in the context of the natural evolution of the disease. To separate these entities from the pattern of outcome would make a clinician rattle off some statistics that can be totally meaningless to a given patient. To be a little more abstract, schizophrenia is a "latent construct," meaning that it is not a concrete diagnostic entity like cancer, pneumonia, or diabetes, whose presenting symptoms can be viewed in the background of histopathology, blood test results, radiological findings, or cultures of biological samples that provide objective evidence of pathology. For these reasons, heterogeneity in the manifestation of the disease and its outcome is a rule than an exception. Narrowing the concept to develop a definition of "nuclear schizophrenia" (as was attempted in the past) does not make the outcome homogenous. This inherently heterogeneous nature of outcome originates, not only from the evolution of the concept of schizophrenia, but also from the natural evolution of the disorder over the years (before, during, and after the onset of illness). This heterogeneity also reflects the innately diverse repertoire of human behavior and emotional reactions. Understanding these aspects and meaningfully translating them to the patient is part of what makes psychiatry an intensely human discipline worth pursuing.

It should be clear now that the outcome of schizophrenia is not as bleak as once thought. About three-fourths of patients can expect to have reasonably good outcomes. Bigger questions concern what difference, if any, that modern treatment makes in altering the course and outcome of schizophrenia. Currently available antipsychotics are effective in treating positive symptoms but only modestly affect the negative symptoms that, to some extent, predict poor outcome. However, antipsychotics and novel drugs in development do not substantially affect the cognitive impairments that contribute considerably to long-term outcome (Buchanan et al., 2011; Meltzer & McGurk, 1999). Thus, novel treatments directed at cognitive impairments and negative symptoms are more likely to favorably affect long-term outcome. Recent advances in psychosocial treatments are showing promise in that direction. Certain forms of cognitive remediation and cognitive enhancement therapies that use computerized cognitive tasks and group therapies have resulted in moderate improvement in cognitive performance at the end of therapies (McGurk, Twamley, Sitzer, McHugo, & Mueser, 2007). Such treatments have further shown that the improvement demonstrated at the end of cognitive enhancement strategies remained sustained at the end of one (Eack, Greenwald, Hogarty, & Keshavan, 2010) and two (Eack et al., 2009) years. Of particular note is the early evidence of possible restitution of some neurobiological systems following some of these therapies (Eack, Hogarty, et al., 2010). There are also ongoing attempts to identify subgroups of schizophrenia patients who may be amenable to specific adjuvant treatments to improve cognitive performance. For example, multiple recent studies note that exposure to the common cold sore virus (herpes simplex virus, type 1) was associated with cognitive impairments (Prasad, Watson, Dickerson, Yolken, & Nimgaonkar, 2012) that improved following supplemental treatment with anti-herpes–specific treatment (Prasad et al., 2013).

The lack of breakthroughs in more effective treatments for schizophrenia and related disorders has paved the path for proposing alternate approaches to investigate the neurobiology of mental disorders without using the DSM framework. One such approach is called the Research Domain Criteria (RDoC), which proposes to examine evidence-based domains at multiple levels; namely, genes, molecules, neural circuits, and so on (Insel, 2014; Insel et al., 2010). Such recent approaches instill further hope for much better outcomes and the fuller realization of recovery from these illnesses.

Self-Learning Questions

1. The Wisconsin Card Sort Test (WCST) is a cognitive task that assesses working memory, attention, and executive functioning. If you did a research study examining the WCST performance of patients with psychotic disorders vs. normal controls, what would you expect to find?
   a. Deficits on the WCST are likely to be present even before a patient developed their first episode of psychosis.
   b. Performance on this test has prognostic relevance for functional outcomes (e.g., ability to work, live independently, etc.), although not as strong as the severity of positive symptoms.
   c. Schizophrenia patients performing much worse than controls, by almost two standard deviations.
   d. A+C are correct
   e. A+B+C are correct

2. Onset of psychotic symptoms in schizophrenia is:
   a. Earlier in males
   b. During adolescence or early adulthood
   c. Often triggered by stressful life events
   d. Often preceded by non-psychotic prodromal symptoms for weeks or months
   e. All of the above

3. You are treating a patient with schizophrenia, and the family asks you about the prognosis. Which of these patient characteristics is *most likely* to portend a worse prognosis?
   a. Acute onset
   b. Amotivation
   c. Female gender
   d. Paranoia

4. A 22-year-old computer programmer recently completed hospital treatment for an acute episode of psychosis. He presented with auditory and visual hallucinations, persecutory delusions, marked mood lability, and loose associations. His symptoms had begun abruptly six weeks previously following a breakup with his girlfriend. Prior to this episode, he had always done well academically and socially. All of the following suggest a good prognosis in his case *except:*

a. Short untreated illness duration
b. Affective symptoms
c. Abrupt onset
d. Male gender

Key Learning Points

- Course and outcome in schizophrenia and related disorders historically has depended on diagnostic conceptualizations, with significant variability even across individuals with exactly the same diagnosis.
- Generally speaking, current outcomes are better than previously thought. Three-quarters of individuals have a good prognosis. Although these illnesses cannot be cured, we know that recovery is possible.
- The best predictors of outcome in schizophrenia are cognitive and negative symptoms (not positive symptoms), along with premorbid functioning, duration of untreated psychosis, and treatment adherence over time.

References

Andreasen, N. C., Carpenter, W. T.Jr., Kane, J. M., Lasser, R. A., Marder, S. R., & Weinberger, D. R. (2005). Remission in schizophrenia: Proposed criteria and rationale for consensus. *American Journal of Psychiatry*, 162(3), 441–449. doi: 10.1176/appi.ajp.162.3.441

Bellack, L. (1948). *Dementia Praecox*. New York: Grune & Stratton.

Buchanan, R. W., Keefe, R. S., Lieberman, J. A., Barch, D. M., Csernansky, J. G., Goff, D. C., et al. (2011). A randomized clinical trial of MK-0777 for the treatment of cognitive impairments in people with schizophrenia. *Biological Psychiatry*, 69(5), 442–449. doi: S0006-3223(10)01053-X [pii] 10.1016/j.biopsych.2010.09.052

Challis, S., Nielssen, O., Harris, A., & Large, M. (2013). Systematic meta-analysis of the risk factors for deliberate self-harm before and after treatment for first-episode psychosis. *Acta Psychiatrica Scandinavica*, 127(6), 442–454. doi: 10.1111/acps.12074

Couture, S. M., Penn, D. L., & Roberts, D. L. (2006). The functional significance of social cognition in schizophrenia: A review. *Schizophrenia Bulletin*, 32(Suppl 1), S44–S63. doi: 10.1093/schbul/sbl029

Eack, S. M., Greenwald, D. P., Hogarty, S. S., Cooley, S. J., DiBarry, A. L., Montrose, D. M., et al. (2009). Cognitive enhancement therapy for early-course schizophrenia: Effects of a two-year randomized controlled trial. *Psychiatric Services*, 60(11), 1468–1476. doi: 10.1176/appi.ps.60.11.1468

Eack, S. M., Greenwald, D. P., Hogarty, S. S., & Keshavan, M. S. (2010). One-year durability of the effects of cognitive enhancement therapy on functional outcome in early schizophrenia. *Schizophrenia Research*, 120(1–3), 210–216. doi: 10.1016/j.schres.2010.03.042

Eack, S. M., Hogarty, G. E., Cho, R. Y., Prasad, K. M., Greenwald, D. P., Hogarty, S. S., et al. (2010). Neuroprotective effects of cognitive enhancement therapy against gray matter loss in early schizophrenia: Results from a 2-year randomized controlled trial. *Archives of General Psychiatry*, 67(7), 674–682. doi: 2010.63 [pii]; 10.1001/archgenpsychiatry.2010.63

Elvevag, B., & Goldberg, T. E. (2000). Cognitive impairment in schizophrenia is the core of the disorder. *Critical Reviews in Neurobiology*, 14(1), 1–21.

Fazel, S., Gulati, G., Linsell, L., Geddes, J. R., & Grann, M. (2009). Schizophrenia and violence: Systematic review and meta-analysis. *PLoS Medicine*, 6(8), e1000120. doi: 10.1371/journal.pmed.1000120

Feinberg, I. (1982). Schizophrenia: Caused by a fault in programmed synaptic elimination during adolescence? *Journal of Psychiatric Research*, 17(4), 319–334.

Frangou, S. (2010). Cognitive function in early onset schizophrenia: A selective review. *Frontiers in Human Neuroscience*, 3, 79. doi: 10.3389/neuro.09.079.2009

Freyhan, F. A. (1955). Course and outcome of schizophrenia. *American Journal of Psychiatry*, 112(3), 161–169.

Golenkov, A., Nielssen, O., & Large, M. (2014). Systematic review and meta-analysis of homicide recidivism and schizophrenia. *BMC Psychiatry*, 14, 46. doi: 10.1186/1471-244X-14-46

Green, M. F., Kern, R. S., Braff, D. L., & Mintz, J. (2000). Neurocognitive deficits and functional outcome in schizophrenia: Are we measuring the "right stuff"? *Schizophrenia Bulletin*, 26(1), 119–136.

Haas, G. L., & Sweeney, J. A. (1992). Premorbid and onset features of first-episode schizophrenia. *Schizophrenia Bulletin*, 18(3), 373–386.

Harding, C. M. (1988). Course types in schizophrenia: An analysis of European and American studies. *Schizophrenia Bulletin*, 14(4), 633–643.

Harding, C. M., Brooks, G. W., Ashikaga, T., Strauss, J. S., & Breier, A. (1987a). The Vermont longitudinal study of persons with severe mental illness, I: Methodology, study sample, and overall status 32 years later. *American Journal of Psychiatry, 144*(6), 718–726.

Harding, C. M., Brooks, G. W., Ashikaga, T., Strauss, J. S., & Breier, A. (1987b). The Vermont longitudinal study of persons with severe mental illness, II: Long-term outcome of subjects who retrospectively met DSM-III criteria for schizophrenia. *American Journal of Psychiatry, 144*(6), 727–735.

Harris, E. C., & Barraclough, B. (1998). Excess mortality of mental disorder. *British Journal of Psychiatry, 173*, 11–53.

Hawton, K., Sutton, L., Haw, C., Sinclair, J., & Deeks, J. J. (2005). Schizophrenia and suicide: Systematic review of risk factors. *British Journal of Psychiatry, 187*, 9–20. doi: 10.1192/bjp.187.1.9

Hegarty, J. D., Baldessarini, R. J., Tohen, M., Waternaux, C., & Oepen, G. (1994). One hundred years of schizophrenia: A meta-analysis of the outcome literature. *American Journal of Psychiatry, 151*(10), 1409–1416.

Insel, T. R. (2014). The NIMH Research Domain Criteria (RDoC) Project: Precision medicine for psychiatry. *American Journal of Psychiatry, 171*(4), 395–397. doi: 10.1176/appi.ajp.2014.14020138

Insel, T. R., Cuthbert, B., Garvey, M., Heinssen, R., Pine, D. S., Quinn, K., et al. (2010). Research domain criteria (RDoC): Toward a new classification framework for research on mental disorders. *American Journal of Psychiatry, 167*(7), 748–751. doi: 10.1176/appi.ajp.2010.09091379

Jaaskelainen, E., Juola, P., Hirvonen, N., McGrath, J. J., Saha, S., Isohanni, M., et al. (2013). A systematic review and meta-analysis of recovery in schizophrenia. *Schizophrenia Bulletin, 39*(6), 1296–1306. doi: 10.1093/schbul/sbs130

Jarbin, H., Ott, Y., & Von Knorring, A. L. (2003). Adult outcome of social function in adolescent-onset schizophrenia and affective psychosis. *Journal of the American Academy of Child and Adolescent Psychiatry, 42*(2), 176–183. doi: 10.1097/00004583-200302000-00011

Joober, R., Rouleau, G. A., Lal, S., Bloom, D., Lalonde, P., Labelle, A., & Benkelfat, C. (2005). Increased prevalence of schizophrenia spectrum disorders in relatives of neuroleptic-nonresponsive schizophrenic patients. *Schizophrenia Research, 77*(1), 35–41. doi: 10.1016/j.schres.2005.01.008

Jorgensen, P. (1994). Course and outcome in delusional disorders. *Psychopathology, 27*(1–2), 79–88.

Kahn, R. S., & Keefe, R. S. (2013). Schizophrenia is a cognitive illness: Time for a change in focus. *Journal of the American Medical Association Psychiatry, 70*(10), 1107–1112. doi: 10.1001/jamapsychiatry.2013.155

Kakela, J., Panula, J., Oinas, E., Hirvonen, N., Jaaskelainen, E., & Miettunen, J. (2014). Family history of psychosis and social, occupational and global outcome in schizophrenia: A meta-analysis. *Acta Psychiatrica Scandinavica, 130*(4), 269–278. doi: 10.1111/acps.12317

Keshavan, M. S., DeLisi, L. E., & Seidman, L. J. (2011). Early and broadly defined psychosis risk mental states. *Schizophrenia Research, 126*(1–3), 1–10. doi: 10.1016/j.schres.2010.10.006

Keshavan, M. S., Haas, G., Miewald, J., Montrose, D. M., Reddy, R., Schooler, N. R., et al. (2003). Prolonged untreated illness duration from prodromal onset predicts outcome in first episode psychoses. *Schizophrenia Bulletin, 29*(4), 757–769.

Kooyman, I., Dean, K., Harvey, S., & Walsh, E. (2007). Outcomes of public concern in schizophrenia. *British Journal of Psychiatry, 50*(Suppl), s29–s36.

Laursen, T. M., Munk-Olsen, T., & Gasse, C. (2011). Chronic somatic comorbidity and excess mortality due to natural causes in persons with schizophrenia or bipolar affective disorder. *PLoS ONE*, *6*(9), e24597. doi: 10.1371/journal. pone.0024597

Laursen, T. M., Munk-Olsen, T., & Vestergaard, M. (2012). Life expectancy and cardiovascular mortality in persons with schizophrenia. *Current Opinion in Psychiatry*, *25*(2), 83–88. doi: 10.1097/YCO.0b013e32835035ca

Laursen, T. M., Nordentoft, M., & Mortensen, P. B. (2014). Excess early mortality in schizophrenia. *Annual Review of Clinical Psychology*, *10*, 425–448. doi: 10.1146/annurev-clinpsy-032813-153657

McGurk, S. R., Twamley, E. W., Sitzer, D. I., McHugo, G. J., & Mueser, K. T. (2007). A meta-analysis of cognitive remediation in schizophrenia. *American Journal of Psychiatry*, *164*(12), 1791–1802.

Meltzer, H. Y., & McGurk, S. R. (1999). The effects of clozapine, risperidone, and olanzapine on cognitive function in schizophrenia. *Schizophrenia Bulletin*, *25*(2), 233–255.

Menezes, N. M., Arenovich, T., & Zipursky, R. B. (2006). A systematic review of longitudinal outcome studies of first-episode psychosis. *Psychological Medicine*, *36*(10), 1349–1362. doi: 10.1017/S0033291706007951

Miller, T. J., McGlashan, T. H., Rosen, J. L., Cadenhead, K., Cannon, T., Ventura, J., et al. (2003). Prodromal assessment with the structured interview for prodromal syndromes and the scale of prodromal symptoms: Predictive validity, interrater reliability, and training to reliability. *Schizophrenia Bulletin*, *29*(4), 703–715.

Modestin, J., Huber, A., Satirli, E., Malti, T., & Hell, D. (2003). Long-term course of schizophrenic illness: Bleuler's study reconsidered. *American Journal of Psychiatry*, *160*(12), 2202–2208.

Murray, R. M., & Lewis, S. W. (1987). Is schizophrenia a neurodevelopmental disorder? *British Medical Journal (Clinical Research Edition)*, *295*(6600), 681–682.

Murray, R. M., O'Callaghan, E., Castle, D. J., & Lewis, S. W. (1992). A neurodevelopmental approach to the classification of schizophrenia. *Schizophrenia Bulletin*, *18*(2), 319–332.

Norman, R. M., Manchanda, R., Malla, A. K., Harricharan, R., & Northcott, S. (2007). The significance of family history in first-episode schizophrenia spectrum disorder. *Journal of Nervous and Mental Disorders*, *195*(10), 846–852. doi: 10.1097/NMD.0b013e318156f8e2

Odegard, O. (1951). Mortality in Norwegian mental hospitals 1926–1941. *Acta Genetica et Statistica Medica*, *2*(2), 141–173.

Opjordsmoen, S., & Retterstol, N. (1993). Outcome in delusional disorder in different periods of time. Possible implications for treatment with neuroleptics. *Psychopathology*, *26*(2), 90–94.

Ostrom, T. M. (1984). The sovereignty of social cognition. In R. S. Wyer & T. K. Srull (Eds.), *Handbook of Social Cognition* (pp. 1–37). Hillsdale, NJ: Lawrence Erlbaum Associates, 1.

Palmer, B. A., Pankratz, V. S., & Bostwick, J. M. (2005). The lifetime risk of suicide in schizophrenia: A reexamination. *Archives of General Psychiatry*, *62*(3), 247–253. doi: 10.1001/archpsyc.62.3.247

Penttila, M., Jaaskelainen, E., Hirvonen, N., Isohanni, M., & Miettunen, J. (2014). Duration of untreated psychosis as predictor of long-term outcome in schizophrenia: Systematic review and meta-analysis. *British Journal of Psychiatry*, *205*(2), 88–94. doi: 10.1192/bjp.bp.113.127753

Pillmann, F., Haring, A., Balzuweit, S., & Marneros, A. (2002). A comparison of DSM-IV brief psychotic disorder with "positive" schizophrenia and healthy controls. *Comprehensive Psychiatry*, *43*(5), 385–392.

Prasad, K. M., Eack, S. M., Keshavan, M. S., Yolken, R. H., Iyengar, S., & Nimgaonkar, V. L. (2013). Antiherpes virus-specific treatment and cognition in schizophrenia: A test-of-concept randomized double-blind placebo-controlled trial. *Schizophrenia Bulletin, 39*(4), 857–866. doi: 10.1093/schbul/sbs040

Prasad, K. M., Watson, A. M., Dickerson, F. B., Yolken, R. H., & Nimgaonkar, V. L. (2012). Exposure to HERPES SIMPLEX VIRUS TYPE 1 and cognitive impairments in individuals with schizophrenia. *Schizophrenia Bulletin*. doi: 10.1093/schbul/sbs046

Robinson, D. G., Woerner, M. G., McMeniman, M., Mendelowitz, A., & Bilder, R. M. (2004). Symptomatic and functional recovery from a first episode of schizophrenia or schizoaffective disorder. *American Journal of Psychiatry, 161*(3), 473–479.

Saha, S., Chant, D., & McGrath, J. (2007). A systematic review of mortality in schizophrenia: is the differential mortality gap worsening over time? *Archives of General Psychiatry, 64*(10), 1123–1131. doi: 10.1001/archpsyc.64.10.1123

Salomon, J. A., Vos, T., Hogan, D. R., Gagnon, M., Naghavi, M., Mokdad, A., et al. (2012). Common values in assessing health outcomes from disease and injury: Disability weights measurement study for the Global Burden of Disease Study 2010. *Lancet, 380*(9859), 2129–2143. doi: 10.1016/S0140-6736(12)61680-8

Strous, R. D., Alvir, J. M., Robinson, D., Gal, G., Sheitman, B., Chakos, M., et al. (2004). Premorbid functioning in schizophrenia: Relation to baseline symptoms, treatment response, and medication side effects. *Schizophrenia Bulletin, 30*(2), 265–278.

Sullivan, H. S. (1994). The onset of schizophrenia. 1927. *American Journal of Psychiatry, 151*(6 Suppl), 134–139.

Warner, R. (2004). *Recovery of Schizophrenia: Psychiatry and Political Economy.* London: Routledge.

Weinberger, D. R. (1987). Implications of normal brain development for the pathogenesis of schizophrenia. *Archives of General Psychiatry, 44*(7), 660–669.

Wyatt, R. J. (1995). Early intervention for schizophrenia: can the course of illness be altered? *Biological Psychiatry, 38*, 1–3.

Yung, A. R., & McGorry, P. D. (1996). The prodromal phase of first-episode psychosis: Past and current conceptualizations. *Schizophrenia Bulletin, 22*(2), 353–370.

Zhang-Wong, J., Beiser, M., Bean, G., & Iacono, W. G. (1995). Five-year course of schizophreniform disorder. *Psychiatry Research, 59*(1–2), 109–117.

Zubin, J., Sutton, S., Salzinger, K., Salzinger, S., Burdock, E. I., & Peretz, D. (1961). A biometric approach to prognosis in schizophrenia. In P. Hoch & J. Zubin (Eds.), *Comparative Epidemiology of Mental Disorders* (pp. 143–203). New York: Grune & Stratton.

Neurobiology
of Schizophrenia

Gil D. Hoftman and Dean F. Salisbury

Introduction

Schizophrenia is a debilitating disorder (or group of disorders) affecting around one percent of the general population. With typical onset of psychosis in late adolescence or young adulthood, and a generally poor prognosis, schizophrenia has lifelong effects on the patient's quality of life. (Please see Chapter 3, "Epidemiology of Schizophrenia," and Chapter 4, "Course, Prognosis, and Outcomes," for greater details.) Understanding the underlying brain changes and dysfunction that lead to schizophrenia is a crucial step towards development of medically and biologically based treatments to alleviate the great suffering caused by this insidious and incapacitating disease and the accompanying stigma. In this chapter, we will discuss the neurobiology of schizophrenia, including in vivo structural volumetric studies and functional studies in living individuals from neuroimaging, including magnetic resonance imaging (MRI) and electroencephalography (EEG), and relevant basic and clinical neuroscience studies relating neural networks, neurotransmitters, and channels. Although psychotic disorders include schizophrenia, schizoaffective, and delusional disorders, we will focus this chapter broadly on schizophrenia, since the sample sizes in most studies have been too small to reliably compare subjects with either schizophrenia or schizoaffective disorder to those with delusional disorder. In addition, the majority of cellular or molecular studies that have examined subjects with schizophrenia and those with schizoaffective disorder found no difference by diagnosis (Eggan et al., 2008; Morris et al., 2008; Eggan et al., 2010; Beneyto et al., 2011; Hoftman et al., 2015; but see Bychkov et al., 2011; Glausier et al., 2015).

Major Points

- Schizophrenia accounts for 1% of the population
- Subtle gray matter changes occur, which only recently have been measured with MRI in vivo

For much of the twentieth century, schizophrenia was conceptualized as a psychological illness, which in many ways mirrored the growth of psychoanalytic perspectives in the early twentieth century. This approach, coupled with the lack of demonstrable pathology in schizophrenia through the 1970s, led to the disease's being termed the "graveyard of neuropathologists" (Plum, 1972). However, the application of in vivo MRI studies of patients shifted the field back towards a neuropsychiatric conceptual framework to find aberrant biological mechanisms within the cortex. In the last 30 years, substantial knowledge of the pathology and pathophysiology of the disorder has come to light, which has changed our understanding of the course and treatment of schizophrenia.

Symptom Clusters

In the 1980s, Andreasen in the United States (e.g., Andreasen & Olsen, 1982) and Crow in the United Kingdom (e.g., Crow, 1982) championed the idea of a two-factor model of schizophrenia: positive and negative symptoms. As discussed in previous chapters, positive symptoms include thoughts and behaviors that are not generally present in healthy individuals, such as paranoia or receiving secret messages from the television. Negative symptoms indicate a lack of a behavior typically seen in healthy individuals, such as a restricted range of nonverbal facial expressions, or reduced motivation and initiative. Liddle (1987) developed an alternative three-factor model that included reality distortion, psychomotor poverty, and disorganization, which are often considered analogous to positive, negative, and cognitive symptom clusters, respectively. The cognitive or disorganization factor refers to problems in ordered, organized thinking and cognitive deficits, such as in working memory. These three factors appear to be the most robust. Although several five-factor models of symptoms and even seven-factor models in schizophrenia have been reported, we will generally speak of the three factors of positive, negative, and cognitive symptoms in relation to pathology and pathophysiology.

As a reminder, positive symptoms include hallucinations (40–70% of patients experience hearing voices), delusions, thought disorder, and affective dysregulation (lability) or flattening. They typically have a waxing and waning course and are variable across episodes, both within and between individuals. Although florid positive symptoms often lead to hospitalization, cognitive ability and negative symptoms are the best predictors of long-term functional outcome. More specifically, verbal memory (medium to large effect), working memory and executive functioning (small to medium effect), and attention/vigilance (small to medium effect) are related to outcome, as are persistent negative symptoms (Green 1996, Green et al. 2000; Gonzalez-Blanch et al., 2010; Fett et al., 2011). Vesterager et al. (2012) showed that working memory performance and negative symptoms predicted functional capacity and real-world functioning at 10 months after first episode. Generally speaking, positive symptoms are relatively well managed by current medications, whereas no standard pharmacological approaches treat negative and cognitive deficits. Hence, to the extent that negative and cognitive problems remain after treatment, their severity plays a significant role in functional outcome in schizophrenia.

Major Points
- Symptoms:
  - Can wax and wane over time (positive)
  - Can also include stable deficits (negative/cognitive)
  - Group reliably into positive, negative, and cognitive factors
- Cognitive deficits and negative symptoms best predict functional outcome.

CT Studies/MRI Studies—Gross Pathology

Schizophrenia has long been associated with enlargement of the ventricles, indicative of a reduction in brain matter volume. This was really the only reliable structural finding until the 1990s, and was demonstrated in patients by using various methods, including pneumo-encephalography (Jacobi & Winkler, 1928), where the cerebrospinal fluid was removed and replaced with air, and a series of X-rays were taken; the first X-ray computed tomography (CT) study of schizophrenia (Johnstone et al., 1976), which reignited the search for structural deficits in schizophrenia; and the first MRI study of schizophrenia (Smith et al., 1984). However, precisely what was reduced in the brain, leading to the enlargement of ventricles, remained unknown. Technological advances in the 1990s in MRI methods gave the spatial resolution necessary detect subtler anatomical changes in schizophrenia.

Studies utilizing structural MRI have yielded several major findings (for further detail, the interested reader is referred to the landmark review of Shenton et al., 2001). Figure 5.1, Panel A, presents MRI images highlighting the major areas of brain gray matter loss in schizophrenia at first hospitalization. Volume reduction is preferential in the medial temporal lobe structures of the limbic system, which includes the amygdala and hippocampus, which are functionally related to memory and emotion. Gray matter loss is also found in the surrounding parahippocampal gyrus. These medial temporal lobe reductions, however, are common to other psychotic disorders, such as bipolar disorder with mania and psychotic features, and thus may not be specific to schizophrenia. Gray matter reductions are also present in the cingulate gyrus, a major interface between limbic and neocortical areas.

Cognitive symptoms have also led researchers to look for volume losses in two specific cortical areas: the frontal lobes, where many of the higher memory, cognitive, emotional, and complex psychomotor planning occurs; and the temporal lobes, specialized for auditory processing and language analysis. In patients with schizophrenia, across the entire brain, there is an approximately 2% gray matter reduction; in the frontal and temporal lobes, gray matter is reduced by about 7% (Nakamura et al., 2007). Although these are relatively small reductions (and indicate the insensitivity of older methods to detect changes), these

A. Major areas of gray matter loss in schizophrenia

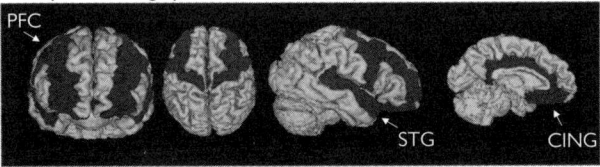

B. Major areas of progressive gray matter loss after first psychosis

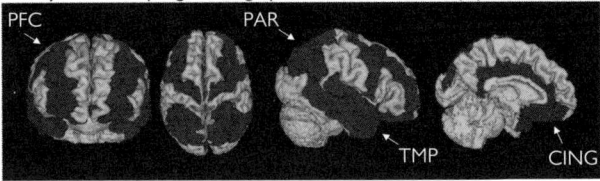

C. Major white matter tract abnormalities in schizophrenia

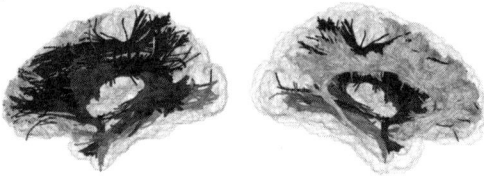

Figure 5.1 *MR imaging of the brain in schizophrenia*: Panel A. At first hospitalization for late adolescent/early adult–onset schizophrenia, gray matter volume reductions are present in many cortical areas, particularly regions that integrate information from other areas. PFC—prefrontal cortex, STG—superior temporal gyrus, CING—cingulate gyrus.

Panel B. Progressive loss also occurs during early disease course, and is greatest in prefrontal, temporal, and parietal heteromodal areas. PFC—prefrontal cortex, PAR—parietal cortex, TMP—temporal cortex, CING—cingulate gyrus.

Panel C. White matter changes are also observed in schizophrenia. Cingulum bundle (light gray), uncinate fasciculus (medium dark gray), arcuate fasciculus (gray), superior longitudinal fasciculus (all three branches—dark gray), inferior longitudinal fasciculus (medium light gray). Corpus callosum not displayed, only for visualization purposes.

Figure 5.1 courtesy of Drs. Martha E Shenton, Johanna Seitz, and Marek Kubicki, Psychiatry NeuroImaging Laboratory, Brigham and Women's Hospital, Harvard Medical School.

gray matter reductions have debilitating effects on the ability of cortical circuits to process information, both in local assemblies and across distributed circuits. In the frontal lobes, the dorso-lateral prefrontal cortex, involved in the flexible use of working memory, shows marked volume reductions. Generally speaking, reductions in frontal lobe volume, including in prefrontal and in medial/orbitofrontal cortex, are associated with increased negative symptoms, cognitive deficits, mood dysregulation, and reward-processing abnormalities. In the temporal lobes, cortical gray matter in the posterior superior temporal gyrus specialized for complex acoustic analysis and language processing is reduced, particularly in the left hemisphere. Temporal lobe gray matter reductions have been associated with increased positive symptoms, including paranoia and delusions, and thought disorder. Lesser reductions have been reported for parietal cortex, typically in the inferior parietal lobule including angular and supramarginal gyri, adjacent to posterior temporal cortex, which perform complex cortical processing.

A useful idea for understanding cortical changes in schizophrenia was proposed by Ross and Pearlson (1996), who suggested that reduction was preferential for heteromodal areas that receive input from many other processing areas in the brain and serve to integrate information across multiple parallel streams. Such heteromodal areas span the frontal, parietal, and temporal lobes, and have large computational demands, which probably rely on a greater number of dendrites and synapses in their local circuitry.

Major Points

- Gray matter loss occurs to a greater degree in heteromodal areas—the areas integrating information from other cortical areas.
- Loss in prefrontal cortex is associated with negative symptoms and cognitive deficits.
- Loss in temporal cortex is associated with positive symptoms and thought disorder.

Other specialized areas of cortex, such as the fusiform gyrus, specialized for face processing, show gray matter volume reductions in schizophrenia, with the loss associated with poorer social functioning. Abnormalities have also been reported for basal ganglia (a major site of action for traditional anti-dopaminergic neuroleptics), in the corpus callosum connecting the hemispheres, the insula, and also for the cerebellum. In summary, however, as a rule of thumb, the major cortical gray matter reductions observed using in vivo MRI occur in the frontal lobe, which correlates with negative symptoms and some cognitive deficits, and in the temporal lobe, which correlates with positive symptoms and other cognitive deficits.

Structural Deficits During Early Disease Course

With the emerging identification of brain pathology in chronically ill subjects in the 1980s and 1990s, researchers focused on first-episode, or more accurately "first-hospitalized," patients to assess which brain changes occurred around the time of the emergence of psychosis. In contrast to the prevailing idea that schizophrenia was caused solely by a static perinatal lesion (see Harrison and Weinberger 2005), it became apparent that the emergence of psychosis was associated with another period of progressive loss of gray matter in the cerebral cortex of patients and a complementary increase in ventricle and sulcal space post-onset. Figure 5.1, Panel B, presents the major areas of progressive gray matter loss following a first hospitalization for schizophrenia. Other brain changes, such as reduced hippocampus volumes, appeared to be present at the time of first psychosis.

When coupled with the evidence that people with schizophrenia had poor premorbid adjustment, including delays in childhood developmental milestones; poorer academic and social school performance; and a demonstrable decline in several domains, including cognitive, social, and occupational functioning, prior to their first "break" from reality, it became apparent that psychosis was not the onset of schizophrenia, but the endpoint of a period of functional decline and subtly increasing pathophysiology, now termed the *prodrome*. The schizophrenia prodrome is a period of active functional decline with the emergence of weak, attenuated psychotic symptoms. When florid psychosis emerges, there is a period of disease progression, with a typical waxing and waning symptom course and a relative lessening of symptom severity over time. However, the decline of social functioning below premorbid levels is often persistent. (For full discussion of this emerging view, please see Chapter 4, "Course, Prognosis, and Outcome in Schizophrenia and Related Disorders.") Whether late-stage schizophrenia is associated with cognitive decline is controversial, although some evidence suggests a slightly greater than normal cognitive decline with aging among older adults with the disorder (Harvey et al., 2006).

In first-hospitalized patients, several groups have identified cortical gray matter changes during the early course of the disorder. In patients with their first episode in young adulthood, the greatest initial deficit was in the left temporal cortex, which showed progressive changes over time, along with bilateral gray matter loss in the temporal and frontal cortices (Hirayasu et al., 2000; Kasai et al., 2003), and in widespread portions of the anterior cingulate gyrus and insula (Asami et al., 2012). In early-onset schizophrenia, Thompson et al. (2001) showed initial reductions in parietal cortex, which spread progressively to temporal and frontal cortices.

In concert, although the exact pattern of cortical changes is not precisely known, these findings suggest that structural changes reflected in cortical gray matter volume loss are present at first hospitalization and continue for at least the early course of the disorder. Significant loss is present in the hippocampus and temporal lobes at first-onset psychosis, with progressive loss in the volume of frontal and temporal cortices, anterior cingulate, inferior parietal lobule, and insula.

Associations between structural loss and symptoms early in disease course appear to follow the same general pattern as in chronically ill schizophrenia; progressive loss in bilateral frontal gray matter and insula, and left inferior parietal lobule are associated with increased negative symptoms, and progressive loss in temporal lobe is associated with increased positive symptoms (such as hallucinations and bizarre delusions), and thought disorder (Asami et al., 2012). Associations between structural loss early in disease course and functional brain activity measures will be described in the next section.

Scant but emerging evidence suggests that this cortical gray matter loss begins in the prodromal phase. It is important to clarify that gray matter losses do not necessarily equate to neuronal death. Note that the number of pyramidal neurons, the main cortical processing units, is not reduced in schizophrenia. Instead, the packing density of cells is increased, suggesting a loss of the gray matter surrounding the pyramidal neurons rather than cell death (Rajkowska et al., 1998; Thune et al., 2001). The leading candidate for this loss is a reduction in dendrites and dendritic spines, leading to the description of the underlying pathology of schizophrenia as *dendrotoxicity* (Olney and Farber, 1995).

Major Points
- Progressive gray matter loss occurs early in the disease course.
- Prefrontal and temporal cortex are preferentially involved.
- Gray matter loss probably reflects reductions of synapses and dendrites rather than neuronal death.

Neurophysiology

The study of neurophysiology has gained increasing importance over the last decade in our understanding of the biological underpinnings of schizophrenia. Several diverse techniques have been used in research to explore neurophysiology. For example, methods based on hemodynamics measure the flow of blood to replenish oxygen supplies in areas of the brain used for specific tasks or in particular states. Positron emission tomography (PET) uses radioactive substances typically attached to sugar or water to track blood flow. Specific chemicals or drugs can be radio-labeled to see where they bind. Functional magnetic resonance imaging (fMRI) detects the slight change in signal caused by oxygenated blood perfusing an area.

In schizophrenia, studies using both methods have shown a relative hypoactivity of anterior areas of the brain in comparison with that of posterior areas. These findings illustrate the general understanding that persons with schizophrenia tend to have deficits in utilizing frontal lobe structures in service of thinking, planning, and memory, and rely more on processing in posterior perceptual integration areas in parietal and temporal cortex. One of the marked problems in schizophrenia revealed by fMRI is reduced function of the dorsolateral prefrontal cortex, an area crucial for attention and working memory. fMRI also demonstrates reduced communication between dorsolateral prefrontal cortex and anterior cingulate cortex, an area integrating habitual and flexible response demands that modulates performance based on errors. fMRI studies have further shown pathophysiology in additional cortical areas. For example, the auditory cortex in the temporal lobe is activated during auditory hallucinations (Dierks et al., 1999), suggesting that the underlying basis for hearing "voices" includes activation of the basic sensory machinery of the brain, although precisely how this occurs remains unknown.

EEG and magnetoencephalography (MEG) measure the activity of cortical neurons, electrical and magnetic, respectively. Because these methods measure the fields of pyramidal cell dendrites, these techniques provide measures of cortical functioning with very high temporal precision, on the order of millisecond, or even sub-millisecond, resolution. In the 1960s, signal averaging techniques were developed so that processing of sights and sounds could be extracted from the EEG. Unlike fMRI, which has tended to examine the frontal lobes and complex behavior like working memory, neurophysiological techniques tend to study more basic sensory and perceptual phenomena. In the late 1960s, it was discovered that anticipating a specific stimulus elicited a brainwave termed the "P300," a positive signal around 300 milliseconds after the stimulus. This was the first objective physiological sign of a cognitive event, and later research determined that P300 was a sensitive index of attention. P300 tasks were quickly applied in schizophrenia research because of the attention problems in the disease. Reductions in P300 are one of the most robust neurophysiological deficits in schizophrenia (see Salisbury et al., 1999), and occur at first hospitalization (Salisbury et al., 1998), and probably in the prodrome as well (van Tricht et al., 2010). P300s normally seen with functional interrogation of the temporal lobe, which can be done by exposing a subject to sound, are reportedly reduced in schizophrenia. This may be considered a trait finding in schizophrenia, as it appears to be stable throughout the lifetime of the disorder. On the other hand, visual P300s induced by occipital lobe activation seem to be more sensitive to state, as they wax and wane with the severity of psychosis. However, while P300 reduction is present robustly in schizophrenia, it is not pathognomonic, as it is observed across many neurological and psychiatric disorders.

P300 is typically evoked by the active detection of an infrequent target stimulus among frequent rare stimuli (Figure 5.2, Panels A & B). Another event-related potential is evoked by stimulus deviance, the mismatch negativity (MMN; Figure 5.2, Panel C). MMN reflects the activity within auditory cortex and is elicited even when sounds are ignored. It probably reflects an initial stage of auditory perception related to a call for an orienting response. This brainwave is highly impaired in chronically ill patients with schizophrenia, but it is relatively unimpaired in first-hospitalized schizophrenia (Salisbury et al., 2002, 2007). MMN indexes cortical gray matter loss during the early course of schizophrenia, and deficits emerge during the first few years in concert with the peri-onset cortical gray matter loss in Heschl's gyrus, a gyrus in the superior temporal plane that contains the primary auditory cortex (Salisbury et al., 2007).

Recent neurophysiological studies have shown that brainwaves related to sensory processing are impaired in schizophrenia. The N100 (a negative brainwave 100 milliseconds after a sound) and P200 (a positive brainwave 200 milliseconds after a

Auditory Event-Related Potentials in First Episode Schizophrenia

A. Oddball Standard and Rare Waveforms

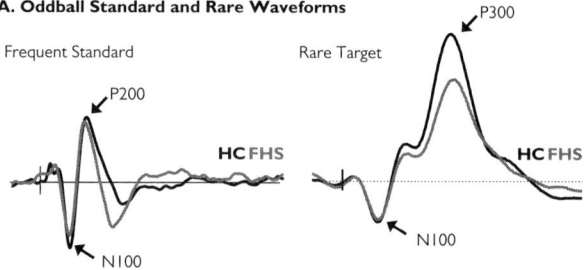

B. Mismatch (MMN) Waveforms

C. 40 Hz Click Train Gamma-Driving SSAEP Waveform

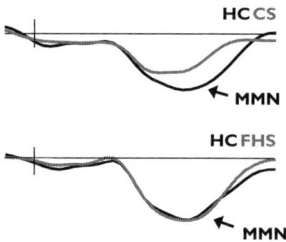

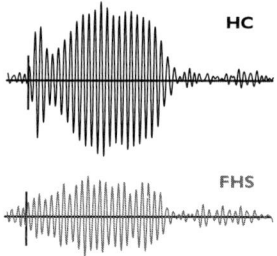

Figure 5.2 *Auditory brainwave deficits in schizophrenia*: Panel A. "Oddball" task deficits. Left tracing responses to standard, frequent tones show reductions of N100 and P200, even at first hospitalization. Right tracings show reductions of the P300 event-related potential to target stimuli.

FHS—first hospitalized schizophrenia, HC—healthy comparison subjects.

Panel B. Mismatch negativity response is impaired in chronic patients (upper tracings) but not at first hospitalization.

CS—chronic schizophrenia, FHS—first hospitalized schizophrenia, HC—healthy comparison subjects.

Panel C. The gamma steady-state auditory evoked potential (SSAEP) shows deficits, even at first hospitalization.

FHS—first hospitalized schizophrenia, HC—healthy comparison subjects.

Waveform tracings courtesy of Salisbury Laboratory, Clinical Neurophysiology Research Laboratory, University of Pittsburgh, Pittsburgh, PA, USA.

sound) are reduced, consistent with the report of hearing problems patients express (Figure 5.2, Panel A). Also known as the "auditory evoked potentials" (AEPs), N100 and P200 reflect a late stage of perception, probably the conscious perception of a sound. The N100 is further reduced when patients are hearing voices, suggesting that portions of auditory cortex are actively responding to the hallucinations. Thus, basic sensory auditory processing is impaired in schizophrenia. Compounding the problem is the fact that sensory and perceptual mechanisms are activated when hallucinations occur, further impairing processing of actual sounds and speech. When one speaks, connections between frontal motor and temporal sensory cortices dampen the N100 response to one's own speech via a so-called corollary discharge; this process appears to be deficient in persons with schizophrenia, and it may contribute to the experience of auditory verbal hallucinations. Other work has suggested that hallucinators have greater impairment in automatic detection of deviance as reflected in MMN.

In the last decade or so, neurophysiologists have focused on brainwave oscillations in schizophrenia. Processing in local circuits is reflected in gamma activity (about 40 Hz and higher), and synchronous firing across cell assemblies is thought to reflect the integration of information across local circuits. Patients with both long-term and first-episode schizophrenia show reductions in task-related gamma activity. For example, when auditory cortex is stimulated by rapid clicks at 40 Hz, patients show reduced ability to process sounds at the brain's optimal rate, in contrast with healthy subjects who show greatest responses at gamma stimulation frequencies (Figure 5.2, Panel C). Gamma deficits have attracted a lot of attention because of their link to basic circuit models of dysfunctional cortex in schizophrenia, in particular the **p**yramidal cell–**i**nter**n**euron–**g**amma or PING model. Long-range communication across cortical areas may be reflected in theta (4–8 Hz) and alpha (8–12 Hz) oscillations, and patients with schizophrenia have reductions in coherent coordinated theta and alpha activity, and fewer interconnected areas than do healthy subjects. Furthermore, alpha activity is reduced by attention, and patients show abnormalities in modulating alpha by attention. Before turning to studies of distributed processing that rely on such long-range communication and integration, we will present more details about the molecular aspects of local circuits.

Major Points

- Sensory and cognitive neurophysiological measures are reduced in schizophrenia.
- Some functions, such as MMN, appear preserved at first break, but become impaired in tandem with progressive gray matter loss.
- The ability of local circuits and long-range distributed circuits to oscillate together in service of information processing and coherent functioning is impaired.

Neurotransmitter Systems and Schizophrenia

Dopamine is a modulatory neurotransmitter long understood to play a critical role in schizophrenia. Four major dopamine pathways have been implicated in the neurobiology of schizophrenia and the side effects of antipsychotic drugs: (1) mesolimbic, (2) mesocortical, (3) nigrostriatal, and (4) tuberoinfundibular. The mesolimbic pathway projects from dopamine-producing neurons in the brainstem to the limbic areas of the brain, especially the human homologue of the nucleus accumbens, which has a central role in reward circuitry. Hyperactivity of the mesolimbic dopamine pathway may underlie some of the positive symptoms of schizophrenia, and a consequence of this pathophysiology could be the faulty association of reward or salience to events. The mesocortical pathway also arises from the brainstem but projects to cortical areas. Negative and cognitive symptoms of schizophrenia may be related to decreased activity in the mesocortical pathway, which could result in reduced dopamine neurotransmission in cortical areas such as the prefrontal cortex. The nigrostriatal pathway projects from the substantia nigra to the basal ganglia, the major site of action of classic antipsychotics, which is thought to be a major site of dopamine-blocking antipsychotics, with side effects that can include rigidity and tardive dyskinesia. The tuberoinfundibular pathway, which projects from the hypothalamus to the anterior pituitary, may also contribute to side effects of antipsychotic medications, such as hyperprolactinemia. Interestingly, there is also an important dopamine circuit modulating eye movement, and abnormalities of dopamine have been indexed by deficits in the ability of individuals to track a target across the visual field. Such deficits in smooth-pursuit eye movements have also been observed in first-episode schizophrenia. Recent work suggests that genetic variants in dopamine influence eye-movement initiation, and those in glutamate affect pursuit maintenance (Lencer et al., 2014).

Glutamate and γ-aminobutyric acid (GABA) are the major excitatory and inhibitory neurotransmitters in the brain, respectively. Glutamate is principally produced by pyramidal neurons (PYR), while GABA is synthesized mainly by local circuit interneurons (GABA neurons). In schizophrenia, alterations in multiple components of the glutamate and GABA systems have been reported in the prefrontal cortex, auditory cortex, and hippocampus, areas critical for cognitive function, social cognition, and positive symptoms. Interestingly, phencyclidine (PCP) and ketamine both block the activity of glutamate at the N-methyl-D-aspartate (NMDA) receptor, and when given to healthy subjects, they can produce psychotic symptoms similar to those observed in schizophrenia. MMN is exquisitely sensitive to NMDA blockade (Javitt et al., 1996; Umbricht et al., 2000). Subjects given ketamine (NMDA-receptor antagonist) show reductions of MMN that correlate with the degree of their drug-induced psychotic symptoms (Umbricht et al., 2000). A recent hypothesis suggests that GABA neuron dysfunction in schizophrenia may result from NMDA-receptor hypofunction in a subset of these neurons; the interested reader is referred to Gonzalez-Burgos & Lewis, 2012).

Serotonin and acetylcholine are modulatory neurotransmitters that have been increasingly implicated in schizophrenia. Like dopamine, serotonin pathways originate in the brainstem and project to multiple brain areas, including the cortex. Similar to glutamate, serotonin can modulate the activity of the dopamine system, and the antagonism of serotonin receptors, especially the serotonin-receptor subtype 2A (5HT2A), might play a role in the actions of atypical antipsychotics. In contrast, acetylcholine is produced mainly by basal forebrain neurons and activates receptors across multiple brain regions that are also sensitive either to nicotine or to muscarine. Nicotinic, but not muscarinic, acetylcholine-receptor dysfunction has been associated with schizophrenia. Recent evidence implicates the α7-containing nicotinic acetylcholine-receptor system in the pathology of schizophrenia. For example, the α7 subunit gene is linked to schizophrenia, and postmortem human studies have found a reduction in the expression of hippocampal α7 receptors in schizophrenia. Interestingly, rates of cigarette smoking in subjects with schizophrenia have been reported to be as high as 90%, compared to 33% in the general population and between 45–70% in patients with other psychiatric diagnoses, leading to the hypothesis that nicotine is treating a fundamental problem in schizophrenia. In schizophrenia, nicotine administration improves working memory and selective attention, whereas withdrawal exacerbates cognitive impairments. In terms of functional associations, acetylcholine and α7 deficits have been associated with a failure to dampen the auditory evoked response to repeated stimuli, the so-called P50-gating response. However,

Table 5.1 Neurotransmitter Systems Disrupted in Schizophrenia

Neurotransmitter	Structure/Function in the CNS	Origin	Targets/Receptors	Basis for Hypothesized Role in Schizophrenia
Dopamine (DA)	Monoamine/ working memory, attention, reward	Brainstem substantia nigra neurons	Cortex, basal ganglia, hypothalamus/ D1–D5	Positive symptom response to dopamine-receptor blockers; PET studies show exaggerated striatal dopamine release in response to amphetamines in people with schizophrenia
Glutamate	Amino acid/critical for excitatory neurotransmission	Pyramidal neurons (PYR); of cortex and other regions	Mainly other PYR in cortex, but also PV neurons/AMPA; NMDA, Kainate, metabotropic glutamate receptors	Phencyclidine and ketamine recapitulate positive, negative, and cognitive symptoms similar to schizophrenia and are NMDA-receptor antagonists; Alterations in glutamate neurotransmission reported in prefrontal cortex and hippocampus in schizophrenia

(continued)

Table 5.1 Continued

Neurotransmitter	Structure/Function in the CNS	Origin	Targets/Receptors	Basis for Hypothesized Role in Schizophrenia
γ-aminobutyric acid (GABA)	Amino acid/critical for inhibitory neurotransmission	Local circuit interneurons; of cortex and other regions	Mainly cell bodies and dendrites of local PYR and GABA neurons in cortex and other regions/$GABA_{A,B}$	Alterations in GABA synthesis and receptors, as well as parvalbumin, which is expressed by a subpopulation of GABA neurons
Serotonin	Monoamine/ implicated in mood regulation	Brainstem raphe nucleus	Cortical cell bodies, dendrites, presynaptic terminals/$5HT_{1-7}$	Can modulate dopamine system; Serotonin 2A receptors blocked by atypical antipsychotics, possibly providing a unique mechanism for antipsychotic efficacy
Acetylcholine (ACh)	Ester of acetic acid and choline/ Increased responsiveness to sensory stimuli, selective attention, working memory	Basal forebrain nucleus	Projects to cortex/ Nicotinic ACh, Muscarinic ACh	Cigarette smoking as high as 90% in people with schizophrenia, compared with 33% in general population; α7 nicotinic ACh-receptor system implicated in pathology of schizophrenia

this response is unlikely to be a useful biomarker as it is relatively less reliable than other functional measures.

Clearly, multiple neurotransmitter systems are implicated in schizophrenia (Table 5.1). Although neurotransmitters and neuromodulators are often referred to as systems—e.g., the dopamine system or the acetylcholine system—processing in the brain involves the coordinated interaction of various neurons linked into small functional units, or local circuits, which in turn communicate over long distances across the brain, termed "distributed circuits."

Major Points

- By blocking dopamine receptors in multiple neural pathways, classic antipsychotics:
  - Alleviate positive symptoms
  - Cause adverse effects
- Dopamine, glutamate, and GABA systems are altered in schizophrenia.
- Studying neurotransmitter systems in the context of specific neural circuits is key for advancing schizophrenia research.

Circuit Models

Neurons in the adult human brain produce as many as 200 trillion connections, forming massively interconnected networks of neuron populations. This staggering interconnectedness allows the brain to perform highly complex functions such as working memory and selective attention.

Dorsolateral prefrontal cortex circuitry, particularly with respect to deficits in working memory, has served as a model for pathophysiology in schizophrenia. PYR account for about 75% of cortical neurons, while GABA neurons account for about 25%. PYR axon terminals target other PYR both in the same and in other brain regions, while local PYR collaterals target GABA neurons, especially subpopulations that express parvalbumin (PV), which in turn inhibit PYR (Figure 5.3). PV neurons can generate action potentials at high rates due to their inherent membrane properties and thus efficiently synchronize PYR populations (Figure 5.3, Panel A). In addition, the PYR GABA-receptor subtypes that are enriched opposite to PV axon terminals have fast decay kinetics, allowing PYR and PV neurons to interact at very high rates, effectively increasing PYR processing speed. PV neurons also furnish highly divergent axonal arbors, with each PV neuron targeting up to hundreds of PYR (Figure 5.3, Panel B).

Recent studies have demonstrated that PV neurons are critical for sculpting the output of PYR in order to generate the gamma oscillations associated with working memory performance (Cardin et al., 2009; Sohal et al., 2009). Recall that gamma activity is thought to reflect local circuit processing, and with respect to working memory, is thought to reflect maintenance of items in memory. Thus, the rhythmic inhibition of PYR by PV neurons appears to be necessary for generating cortical gamma band oscillations. In pyramidal-interneuron-gamma (PING) neural circuit models, the presence of PYR reciprocally connected with GABA interneurons (for example, PV neurons) results in a stable generation of gamma oscillation frequency. In this model, fast excitation (PYR activity) and delayed feedback inhibition (inhibitory PV neuron inputs to PYR somas and proximal dendrites) alternate, and with the appropriate strength of excitation and inhibition, they create a prolonged cyclical behavior. In support of the PING model, weakening the PYR–PV neuron connection by knocking down glutamate receptors on PV neurons results in weaker gamma oscillations. In schizophrenia, a hypothesized disruption in the balance between excitation and inhibition is

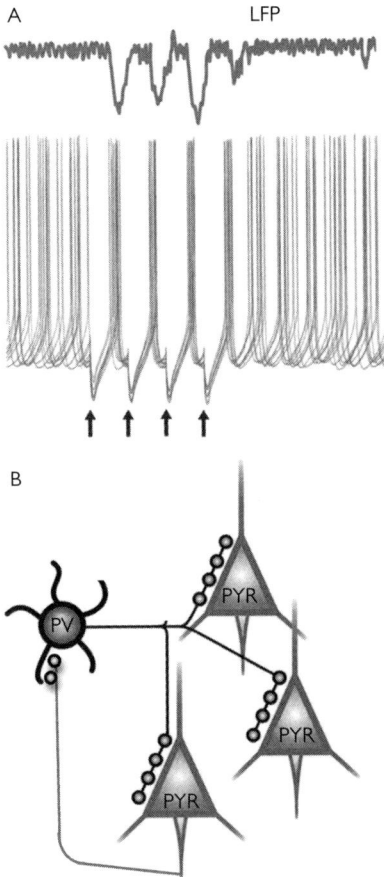

Figure 5.3 *Parvalbumin-containing GABA neurons (PV neurons) synchronize the activity of pyramidal cell populations*: Panel A. Dark gray tracing represents recording of local field potentials (LFP) generated by PV neuron connections onto pyramidal cells. Light gray trace represents recording of action potential spikes from a population of pyramidal cells. Black arrows show synchronized spikes recorded from pyramidal cells. Note that synchronization occurs shortly after LFPs.
Panel B. Schematic diagram showing one PV neuron (circular cell with black outline) sending divergent connections to three pyramidal neurons (PYR; triangular cells with gray outline) and one PYR providing excitatory input to that PV neuron.
Figure modified from Gonzalez-Burgos & Lewis (2008).

the current focus of active investigations. For example, reciprocal excitatory connections in pyramidal neurons located in the prefrontal cortical superficial layers are important for working memory function (Arnsten et al., 2012). In schizophrenia, lower dendritic spine density is observed in these cells (Garey et al., 1998; Glantz & Lewis, 2000), leading to the hypothesis that the balance between excitation and inhibition is altered in schizophrenia.

Given the increasingly recognized importance of PYR–PV neuron connectivity for gamma oscillation activity and cognition, two main hypotheses have been proposed to account for lower GABA-synthesizing enzyme levels in PV neurons in schizophrenia. One posits that PV neurons are primarily affected, resulting in dysfunction leading to PYR disinhibition; while the other argues that PV-innervating PYR neurons represent the primary pathology. According to the second hypothesis, fewer dendritic spines on cortical layer 3 PYR, and thus less excitatory input to these neurons, would result in lower activity (reviewed in Lewis et al., 2012). In turn, these hypoactive cells would produce lower excitatory local network activity, resulting in a homeostatic downregulation of inhibition, measured in part as a decrease in GABA-synthesizing enzymes in PV neurons (reviewed in Lewis et al., 2012). The resulting reduction of inhibition would partially restore the balance between excitation and inhibition, although at a lower set point and perhaps with more limited dynamic range. Further experiments are needed to determine whether primary deficits in PV neurons or in PYR neurons that innervate PV neurons provide the most compelling models for these alterations.

One popular molecular hypothesis posits that NMDA-receptor hypofunction on PV neurons results in disinhibition of pyramidal cells that leads to gamma band oscillatory circuit deficits and consequent cognitive dysfunction in schizophrenia. Recent evidence suggests this model may not be entirely accurate. For example, animal physiology experiments show a large contribution of α-amino-3-hydroxy-5-methyl-4-isoxazolepropionic acid (AMPA)-receptor current and negligible NMDA-receptor current recorded from PV neurons. PV neural control of PYR activity does contribute to gamma oscillations and other rhythmic patterns of cortical network activity crucial for local processing, but other GABA neuron subpopulations also contribute to gamma oscillations. In addition, abnormalities in NMDA receptors located in pyramidal neurons and in somatostatin (SST)- and cholecystokinin (CCK)-containing GABA interneurons (Benneyworth et al., 2011; Tatard-Leitman et al., 2015) suggest a more complex pathophysiology. Thus cognitive deficits in schizophrenia can arise from disturbances in many sources of synaptic inhibition, resulting in alteration of many types of cortical network activity.

Additional circuit models of neural dysfunction in schizophrenia emphasize non-cortical structures like the limbic system, basal ganglia, and thalamus (see reviews by Meador-Woodruff et al., 2003; Lisman et al., 2008; Ferrarelli & Tononi, 2010; Simpson et al., 2010). Integrating the contribution of each brain region to cognitive dysfunction in schizophrenia remains a challenge actively pursued by research laboratories around the world that may help clarify some of the clinical heterogeneity observed in schizophrenia. Finally, given that schizophrenia is increasingly recognized as a disorder of neurodevelopment (Insel, 2010), understanding the mechanisms of PYR and PV neuron development and how other neurotransmitters and modulators affect them is a critical research priority.

Additional neuronal subtypes might also skew excitatory glutamate and inhibitory GABA balance (Table 5.2). The endogenous cannabinoids, which are lipids that have structural features similar to those of the principal psychoactive component of marijuana (Δ^9-THC), block GABA-ergic release from CCK-containing basket cell inhibitory afferents to the PYR proximal dendrites and may be elevated in schizophrenia (Leweke et al., 1999, but cf. Eggan et al., 2008, regarding reduced cannabinoid 1 receptor [CB1R] expression). Glutamic acid decarboxylase 67 (GAD67), the synaptic GABA transporter, and D-serine gene expression are reduced (Coyle et al., 2010). Several other mechanisms affect glutamate–GABA imbalance, including alterations in SST neurons (Morris et al., 2008; Beneyto et al., 2011; Fung et al., 2010; Beneyto et al., 2012).

Markers of astrocyte function, which regulate glutamate in the synaptic cleft, are altered in schizophrenia. Cell cultures deficient in astrocytes not only show fewer synapses, but also are 100 times more susceptible to glutamate toxicity (Harris, 2001). Antagonists at the NMDA receptor such as PCP induce an interleukin-6 anti-inflammatory response that activates production of superoxide, in turn leading to selective dysfunction of PV neurons (Behrens et al., 2008). Increased expression levels of the

Table 5.2 Cortical Neuronal Subtypes Implicated in Cognitive Dysfunction in Schizophrenia

Cortical Cell Type	Hypothesized Receptor Alterations	Endogenous Receptor Ligand	Exogenous Receptor Ligand*	Proposed Circuit Function	Hypothesized Circuit Dysfunction
PYR neurons	NMDA (glutamate receptor) GABRA (GABA receptor)	Glutamate GABA	*NMDA blockers (PCP, ketamine)* Benzodiazepines (valium)	Integrating signals for output to local and distant sites	Reduced excitatory drive possibly contributing to dendritic spine loss
CCK basket neurons	Cannabinoid 1 (CB1)	Endocannabinoids (2-AG, anandamide)	*Tetrahydrocanna-binol (THC) from marijuana*	Fine-tuning local modulatory signals	Disrupted integration of modulatory signals
PV basket neurons	Mu-opioid	Opioids (enkephalin, met-enkephalin)	Opiates (morphine)	Timed excitation and inhibition synchronizes PYR neurons	Disruption of PYR neural synchrony and oscillations
SST neurons	GABRA	GABA	Benzodiazepines (valium)	Modulates activity at PYR neuron dendrites	Currently unknown

*Italicized ligands recapitulate symptoms that resemble schizophrenia in humans.

mu-opioid receptor mRNA in PV neurons have been reported in schizophrenia, and the mu-opioid receptor both decreases PV cell activity and decreases release of GABA from PV axon terminals (Lupica, 1995; Glickfeld et al., 2008; Volk et al., 2012). Thus, many processes converge on the GABA and glutamate balance of local cortical circuits. The findings of lower dendritic spine density and lower presynaptic glutamate synaptic markers within cortically projecting PYR in schizophrenia suggest a reduction in excitatory drive. These findings, together with alterations in markers of GABA neurotransmission such as lower GABA synthesis in PV neurons, lower detectability of immunoreactive GABA inputs to PYR (Lewis et al., 2001; Volk et al., 2002), and dysfunction of the endogenous cannabinoid system (Eggan et al., 2008), suggest that glutamate–GABA imbalance through currently unknown mechanisms (but perhaps related to astrocyte dysfunction, oxidative stress, and/or immune system dysfunction) leads to abnormalities in the synchronization of neural population activity and perhaps alterations in cortical gamma oscillations.

Since the brain relies on precise yet dynamic connections between neurons for proper function, disruptions in specific connections can have devastating functional consequences and might underlie the clinical features of schizophrenia. On the other hand, the remarkable plasticity of these connections offers the possibility that these disruptions could also be ameliorated if identified early and targeted specifically. Studies of local circuit pathophysiology could allow for the development of novel pharmacological interventions. In line with the circuit models described, Lewis et al. (2008) hypothesized that reduced GABA signaling from PV neurons to PYR contributed to prefrontal cortex (PFC)-dependent cognitive dysfunction via a deficit in gamma synchronization. Merck compound MK-0777, a selective $GABA_A$-receptor $\alpha2/\alpha3$ subunit allosteric modulator, was tested in 15 subject pairs (subjects in control and schizophrenia groups matched for age and gender) to attempt to normalize PV–PYR signaling. MK-0777-treated individuals with schizophrenia showed a significant improvement over placebo in a cognitive task over time and an increase in PFC gamma oscillation power. The small sample size clearly requires replication and extension in larger clinical trials, but this study supports the concept that disturbances in induced gamma oscillations underlie deficits in cognitive tasks in schizophrenia.

Major Points

- The **P**yramidal-**I**nter**N**euron **G**amma (PING) model proposes that interconnected PYR and PV neurons are critical for gamma activity.
- Multiple neural circuits may be disrupted in schizophrenia, partially explaining clinical heterogeneity.
- Proof-of-principle interventions targeting specific neural circuits have improved cognitive control and gamma oscillations in schizophrenia subjects.

Distributed Processing and Connectivity

In the last decade, neuroimaging in schizophrenia has become less focused on describing deficits in one cortical area subserving a specific function, and more focused on describing patterns of pathophysiology across dynamic systems involving several interconnected cortical areas. Using fMRI, patterns of correlated activation of areas either on task or at rest have identified several systems that appear to form functional networks. The default network, which is active when the brain is awake but quiescent, a frontal-parietal network, a cingular-opecular network, and a cortico-cerebellar network have all been identified using fMRI. Persons with schizophrenia tend to have weaker connectivity in these networks, although this is not a consistent finding. As task processing demands increase, persons with schizophrenia tend to show less interconnectivity between networks, particularly between the frontal-parietal network thought to reflect cognitive control and other networks. There is evidence that they do not suppress the default network activity while on task either. Thus, active information processing systems are not fully engaged, the default mode is not fully suppressed, and cognitive control is not fully exerted.

Another way to assess functional connectivity is to examine how strongly individual brain areas are interconnected. Consistent with the findings of relative hypofrontality in hemodynamic studies, individuals with schizophrenia tend to show relative hypoconnectivity of the prefrontal cortex, which may be correlated with increased psychopathology, and relative hyperconnectivity of posterior areas. Although the idea that schizophrenia is characterized by disconnection across the brain is well established, it is becoming increasingly apparent that abnormal hyperconnectivity is also present in the syndrome.

Structurally, studies using diffusion tensor imaging examine the white matter tracts that connect cortical areas. As shown in Figure 5.1, Panel C, many of the major white matter bundles connecting different cortical areas of the brain are impaired in schizophrenia. Abnormalities have been observed in the tracts that connect prefrontal cortex that correlate with negative symptoms, impulsiveness, and aggressiveness; and between white matter deficits in cingulum bundle and executive function errors; and between uncinate fasciculus connecting PFC with temporal lobe with verbal memory deficits. Structural connections between frontal cortex (Broca's area) and temporal cortex (Wernicke's area) in the later superior parietal fasciculus and arcuate fasciculus have been shown to be *larger* than normal in patients with auditory hallucinations, while smaller than normal in patients without them. A similar finding in white matter connectivity was observed between the left and right hemispheres. This raises the intriguing possibility that hallucinations may be due to hyperconnectivity of auditory and language areas.

Major Points

- Schizophrenia is associated with less coherent distributed processing and connectivity.
- It's not just disconnectivity; some areas show hyperconnectivity; for example, between Broca's and Wernicke's areas in hallucinators.

In a review of fMRI-based functional connectivity studies of auditory verbal hallucinations in schizophrenia, Hoffman and Hampson (2012) proposed a distributed cortico-striatal language circuit comprising Wernicke's area (temporal), the inferior frontal gyrus, and the putamen. Patients with hallucinations showed increased functional connectivity between these areas, and the authors speculated that the putamen played a role in whether auditory activity was consciously detected as an external event, such that the hyperconnectivity between the putamen and Wernicke's areas led to auditory verbal hallucinations. Of note as a potential new therapy for treatment of hallucinations, stimulation of the temporoparietal junction using transcranial magnetic stimulation (TMS) and direct current stimulation (DCS) has been shown to reduce intractable auditory hallucinations, probably by down-regulating spurious activity in the left temporal Wernicke's area.

Heritability and Genetics

Evidence from twin, family, and adoption studies has shown that the etiology of schizophrenia has an appreciable genetic component. For example, monozygotic (MZ) "identical" twins share 100% of their genes and have a higher rate of concordance (i.e., both twins having disease) for schizophrenia than dizygotic (DZ) "fraternal" twins who share 50% of their genes. However, both monozygotic twins are diagnosed with schizophrenia only 40–60% of the time, suggesting that environmental factors contribute to the disease pathogenesis. Adoption studies have estimated that children adopted into a "healthy" family who have a biological parent with schizophrenia still have a roughly 10% risk of developing the disorder, compared to a 1% risk in the general population. Together with first-degree sibling studies, these investigations have led to high heritability estimates of 70% or ~0.7, indicating that roughly 70% of the risk for schizophrenia is genetic. However, there is evidence against simple Mendelian inheritance, as around 60% of individuals diagnosed with schizophrenia have neither a first- nor a second-degree relative with the illness.

In a structural MRI study of monozygotic and dizygotic twins, Cannon and colleagues (2002) correlated gray matter volumes between healthy individuals, and between individuals discordant for schizophrenia. Such a strategy allowed the separation of gray matter deficits associated with genetic similarity (MZ > DZ) from changes associated with disease-specific processes (discordant MZ twin differences). Healthy MZ twins showed generally high correlations in gray matter volumes across the cortex, in contrast to healthy DZ twins, who only showed high volume correlations in visual and superior parietal gray matter volumes. Genetic liability to schizophrenia mapped onto deficits primarily in the dorsolateral prefrontal cortex, frontal pole, and temporal pole (connected to prefrontal cortex via the uncinate fasciculus). Of primary importance, discordant MZ twins showed disease-specific gray matter volume differences in dorsolateral prefrontal cortex, superior temporal gyrus, and superior parietal lobule, once again revealing heteromodal areas of cortex as particularly susceptible in the disease. Greater frontal and temporal loss was associated with greater negative symptoms, and to a lesser degree with greater positive symptoms, while cognitive deficits were associated with greater loss in all three heteromodal areas, and visual memory deficits were associated with temporal and parietal loss. The same group (Ahveninen et al., 2006) examined P50, N100, and MMN on a passive task, and reported that within the context of all three responses' being impaired in schizophrenia, their discordant twins showed reductions of P50 and N100, but not of MMN. Furthermore, the deficit on discordant twins was greater for MZ than DZ twins, further lending credence to these measures as sensitive to genetic similarity.

Using structural equation modeling on twin and family members, Hall and colleagues (2006, 2011) showed high heritability in schizophrenia for P300 amplitude and latency, P50 gating, and for the early auditory gamma band response, a small burst of gamma activity observed between 50 and 100 milliseconds after a sound. P3 amplitude, P3 latency and the early gamma response, and P50 gating appeared to assess relatively independent genetic contributions, speculatively associated with different genetic risk factors. By contrast, Hall et al. (2007) suggested that MMN showed a substantial environmental component and was significantly associated with schizophrenia only when the highest schizophrenia heritability estimates were used. Thus, several of the neurophysiological measures discussed appear to be viable intermediate endophenotypes, or measures that reflect the physiological consequences of some specific genetic risk variants for schizophrenia.

Major Points

- Some gray matter deficits in polar cortex appear to be heritable.
- Prefrontal and temporal cortex gray matter loss appear to be disease specific.
- Neurophysiological measures are heritable biomarkers, and can provide clues about underlying genetic risk factors.

Genome-wide association studies (GWAS) suggest that an accumulation of risk alleles at many loci can result in the schizophrenia syndrome. In fact, a large study in 2014 reported 168 risk genes at 108 independent loci. Rare structural variants, including 22q11 deletions and 1:11 chromosomal translocations, have also been strongly associated with schizophrenia. In addition, microdeletions or microduplications (copy number variants, or CNVs) have recently been reported to substantially increase the risk for schizophrenia. Despite these recent exciting advances in genotyping methods, the combination of the many genetic susceptibility variants still leaves the majority of schizophrenia heritability unexplained. Still, although many candidate genetic risk variants have been identified, precisely how they map onto structural pathology and functional pathophysiology remain to be determined.

Conclusion

Schizophrenia is associated with subtle yet profoundly impactful reductions of cortical gray matter, which appear to be greatest in higher-order cortical areas. These brain regions, which receive inputs from many other areas, perform the most sophisticated types of processing, and comprise the heteromodal areas in the frontal, temporal, and parietal cortices. Generally speaking, such gray matter loss is associated with increased negative symptoms (frontal), positive symptoms (temporal), and cognitive symptoms (frontal, parietal, and temporal). While the heteromodal areas show the greatest volume changes in in vivo measures, it is likely that the basic cellular deficit is ubiquitous across many regions within the brain. Because heteromodal areas have longer dendrites and more synapses, it is possible that dendrotoxic effects appear greatest there. Still, cortical loss continues progressively during the early course of the disorder and impinges on the rest of the cortical mantle, including the sensory cortex. The basic deficit probably results in an imbalance of excitatory glutamate and inhibitory GABA, in turn perhaps linked to deficits of PYR function. These deficits in PYR excitation, either intrinsic to PYR or from extrinsic inputs to PYR, could lead to a failure of PYR cells to oscillate properly at gamma frequencies in the service of local circuit processing. It is not known what key gene-by-environment interactions lead to the disease-specific gray matter loss that may contribute to schizophrenia.

Structural and functional cortical deficits are associated with abnormalities of neurophysiological measures. P50, N100, P300, and gamma activity all appear to be sensitive to the disease process and sensitive to largely independent underlying genetic risk factors. These measures, recorded in vivo from individuals and situated between the gross structural measures of MRI and molecular measures of post-mortem work and animal models, provide important tools for understanding not only the system-level pathology and pathophysiology of schizophrenia, but the progressive and dynamic course of the disorder's increasing pathology. The goal of much current research is to identify persons who will develop schizophrenia as early as possible (hopefully prior to the emergence of psychosis in the prodromal stage) and prevent the progressive gray matter loss central to the disease's debilitating effects. However, to halt this cortical gray matter loss, we must understand the basic mechanisms of its pathophysiology, so as to develop diagnostic criteria based on this pathophysiology to inform the implementation of evidence-based interventions targeted to rational biochemical or physiological targets (the interested reader is referred to Van Haren et al., 2012).

Self-Learning Questions

1. Novel approaches to treating schizophrenia have emerged from the translational neuroscience paradigm, where a better understanding of pathophysiology can inform clinical care. One approach has been to use GABA-A alpha-2 agonists to enhance gamma band synchronicity in the dorsolateral prefrontal cortex. What feature of schizophrenia, strongly linked to overall outcome, has been shown to improve from this kind of intervention?
   a. Cognitive symptoms (working memory/attention)
   b. Impulsivity symptoms (aggression/suicide)
   c. Negative symptoms (amotivation/alogia)
   d. Positive symptoms (delusions/hallucinations)

2. What is the most likely neuroradiological abnormality that might be found if you imaged the brain of someone with schizophrenia?
   a. Agenesis of the corpus callosum
   b. Enlarged prefrontal cortex
   c. Ventriculomegaly
   d. White matter hyperintensities

3. According to the "dopamine hypothesis," the positive symptoms in schizophrenia result from an excess of dopaminergic neurotransmission in which brain pathway?
   a. Mesolimbic
   b. Nigrostriatal
   c. Tuberoinfundibular
   d. None of the above

4. Electrophysiological findings have helped shed light on aberrant circuitry in schizophrenia. Which statement is most accurate about such observations?
   a. Gamma-band oscillations have been found to be centered around the occipital cortex and seem to closely relate to visual hallucinations.
   b. Mismatch negativity (MMN) worsens over the course of illness, and is tied to gray matter loss.
   c. The N100 wave has been critical to rethinking the previously accepted PING model of brain circuitry in schizophrenia, which has now been abandoned.
   d. Post-stimulus P300 waves on EEG are fairly specific to schizophrenia and have begun to be used as a marker of prodromal illness.

Key Learning Points

- Schizophrenia is characterized by progressive gray matter loss beginning early in the disease course, reflecting reductions of synapses and dendrites (not cell death); areas for greatest loss correlate closely with positive (temporal cortex) and negative/cognitive (prefrontal cortex) symptoms.
- Many sensory and cognitive neurophysiological functions such as mismatch negativity (MMN) become impaired over the course of illness, and these cognitive deficits seem to be particularly linked to the inability of circuits to oscillate together (gamma band), which reduces information processing efficiency.
- The Pyramidal-InterNeuron Gamma (PING) model proposes that interconnected pyramidal and parvalbumin neurons determine gamma activity; interventions targeting these circuits improve cognitive control.
- Such neurophysiological measures are heritable biomarkers and may provide clues about underlying genetic risk factors.
- Several neurotransmitter systems (dopamine, glutamate, GABA) are altered in schizophrenia, with dopamine excess linked to positive symptoms, alleviated by dopamine-blocking antipsychotics.

References

Ahveninen, J., Jääskeläinen, I. P., Osipova, D., Huttunen, M. O., Ilmoniemi, R. J., Kaprio, J., et al. (2006). Inherited auditory-cortical dysfunction in twin pairs discordant for schizophrenia. *Biological Psychiatry*, 60(6), 612–620.

Andreasen, N. C., & Olsen, S. (1982). Negative v. positive schizophrenia: Definition and validation. *Archives of General Psychiatry*, 39(7), 789–794.

Arnsten, A. F., Wang, M. J., & Paspalas, C. D. (2012). Neuromodulation of thought: Flexibilities and vulnerabilities in prefrontal cortical network synapses. *Neuron*, 76(1), 223–239.

Asami, T., Bouix, S., Whitford, T. J., Shenton, M. E., Salisbury, D. F., & McCarley, R. W. (2012). Longitudinal loss of gray matter volume in patients with first-episode schizophrenia: DARTEL automated analysis and ROI validation. *Neuroimage*, 59(2), 986–996.

Behrens, M. M., Ali, S. S., & Dugan, L. L. (2008). Interleukin-6 mediates the increase in NADPH-oxidase in the ketamine model of schizophrenia. *The Journal of Neuroscience*, 28(51), 13957–13966.

Beneyto, M., Abbott, A., Hashimoto, T., & Lewis, D. A. (2011). Lamina-specific alterations in cortical GABAA receptor subunit expression in schizophrenia. *Cerebral Cortex*, 21(5), 999–1011.

Beneyto, M., Morris, H. M., Rovensky, K. C., & Lewis, D. A. (2012). Lamina- and cell-specific alterations in cortical somatostatin receptor 2 mRNA expression in schizophrenia. *Neuropharmacology*, 62(3), 1598–1605.

Benneyworth, M. A., Roseman, A. S., Basu, A. C., & Coyle, J. T. (2011). Failure of NMDA receptor hypofunction to induce a pathological reduction in PV-positive GABAergic cell markers. *Neuroscience Letters*, 488(3), 267–271.

Bychkov, E. R., Ahmed, M. R., Gurevich, V. V., Benovic, J. L., & Gurevich, E. V. (2011). Reduced expression of G protein-coupled receptor kinases in schizophrenia but not in schizoaffective disorder. *Neurobiology of Disease*, 44(2), 248–258.

Cannon, T. D., Thompson, P. M., van Erp, T. G., Toga, A. W., Poutanen, V. P., Huttunen, M., et al. (2002). Cortex mapping reveals regionally specific patterns of genetic and disease-specific gray-matter deficits in twins discordant for schizophrenia. *Proceedings of the National Academy of Sciences*, 99(5), 3228–3233.

Cardin, J. A., Carlén, M., Meletis, K., Knoblich, U., Zhang, F., Deisseroth, K., et al. (2009). Driving fast-spiking cells induces gamma rhythm and controls sensory responses. *Nature*, 459(7247), 663–667.

Coyle, J. T., Balu, D., Benneyworth, M., Basu, A., & Roseman, A. (2010). Beyond the dopamine receptor: Novel therapeutic targets for treating schizophrenia. *Dialogues in Clinical Neuroscience*, 12(3), 359.

Crow, T. J. (1982). Two syndromes in schizophrenia? *Trends in Neurosciences*, 5, 351–354.

Dierks, T., Linden, D. E., Jandl, M., Formisano, E., Goebel, R., Lanfermann, H., et al. (1999). Activation of Heschl's gyrus during auditory hallucinations. *Neuron*, 22(3), 615–621.

Eggan, S. M., Hashimoto, T., & Lewis, D. A. (2008). Reduced cortical cannabinoid 1 receptor messenger RNA and protein expression in schizophrenia. *Archives of General Psychiatry*, 65(7), 772–784.

Eggan, S. M., Stoyak, S. R., Verrico, C. D., & Lewis, D. A. (2010). Cannabinoid CB1 receptor immunoreactivity in the prefrontal cortex: Comparison of schizophrenia and major depressive disorder. *Neuropsychopharmacology*, 35(10), 2060–2071.

Ferrarelli, F., & Tononi, G. (2011). The thalamic reticular nucleus and schizophrenia. *Schizophrenia Bulletin*, *37*(2), 306–315.

Fett, A. K. J., Viechtbauer, W., Penn, D. L., van Os, J., & Krabbendam, L. (2011). The relationship between neurocognition and social cognition with functional outcomes in schizophrenia: A meta-analysis. *Neuroscience and Biobehavioral Reviews*, *35*(3), 573–588.

Fung, S. J., Webster, M. J., Sivagnanasundaram, S., Duncan, C., Elashoff, M., & Weickert, C. S. (2010). Expression of interneuron markers in the dorsolateral prefrontal cortex of the developing human and in schizophrenia. *American Journal of Psychiatry*, *167*(12), 1479–1488.

Garey, L. J., Ong, W. Y., Patel, T. S., Kanani, M., Davis, A., Mortimer, A. M., et al. (1998). Reduced dendritic spine density on cerebral cortical pyramidal neurons in schizophrenia. *Journal of Neurology, Neurosurgery and Psychiatry*, *65*(4), 446–453.

Glantz, L. A., & Lewis, D. A. (2000). Decreased dendritic spine density on prefrontal cortical pyramidal neurons in schizophrenia. *Archives of General Psychiatry*, *57*(1), 65–73.

Glausier, J. R., Kimoto, S., Fish, K. N., & Lewis, D. A. (2015). Lower glutamic acid decarboxylase 65-kDa isoform messenger RNA and protein levels in the prefrontal cortex in schizoaffective disorder but not schizophrenia. *Biological Psychiatry*, *77*(2), 167–176.

Glickfeld, L. L., Atallah, B. V., & Scanziani, M. (2008). Complementary modulation of somatic inhibition by opioids and cannabinoids. *The Journal of Neuroscience*, *28*(8), 1824–1832.

González-Blanch, C., Perez-Iglesias, R., Pardo-García, G., Rodríguez-Sánchez, J. M., Martínez-García, O., Vázquez-Barquero, J. L., et al. (2010). Prognostic value of cognitive functioning for global functional recovery in first-episode schizophrenia. *Psychological Medicine*, *40*(06), 935–944.

Gonzalez-Burgos, G., & Lewis, D. A. (2008). GABA neurons and the mechanisms of network oscillations: Implications for understanding cortical dysfunction in schizophrenia. *Schizophrenia Bulletin*, *34*(5), 944–961.

Gonzalez-Burgos, G., & Lewis, D. A. (2012). NMDA receptor hypofunction, parvalbumin-positive neurons, and cortical gamma oscillations in schizophrenia. *Schizophrenia Bulletin*, *38*(5), 950–957.

Green, M. F. (1996). What are the functional consequences of neurocognitive deficits in schizophrenia? *The American Journal of Psychiatry*, *153*(3), 321.

Green, M. F., Kern, R. S., Braff, D. L., & Mintz, J. (2000). Neurocognitive deficits and functional outcome in schizophrenia: are we measuring the "right stuff"?. *Schizophrenia bulletin*, *26*(1), 119.

Hall, M. H., Rijsdijk, F., Picchioni, M., Psych, M. R. C., Schulze, K., Ettinger, U., et al. (2007). Substantial shared genetic influences on schizophrenia and event-related potentials. *The American Journal of Psychiatry*, *164*(5), 804–812.

Hall, M. H., Taylor, G., Sham, P., Schulze, K., Rijsdijk, F., Picchioni, M., et al. (2011). The early auditory gamma-band response is heritable and a putative endophenotype of schizophrenia. *Schizophrenia Bulletin*, *37*(4), 778–787.

Hall, M. H., Schulze, K., Rijsdijk, F., Picchioni, M., Ettinger, U., Bramon, E., et al. (2006). Heritability and reliability of P300, P50 and duration mismatch negativity. *Behavior Genetics*, *36*(6), 845–857.

Harris, K. M. (2001). Dendritic spines. *eLS*. Wiley Online Library, DOI: 10.1038/npg.els.0000093.

Harrison, P. J., & Weinberger, D. R. (2005). Schizophrenia genes, gene expression, and neuropathology: On the matter of their convergence. *Molecular Psychiatry*, *10*(1), 40–68.

Harvey, P. D., Reichenberg, A., & Bowie, C. R. (2006). Cognition and aging in psychopathology: Focus on schizophrenia and depression. *Annual Review of Clinical Psychology, 2*, 389–409.

Hirayasu, Y., McCarley, R. W., Salisbury, D. F., Tanaka, S., Kwon, J. S., Frumin, M., et al. (2000). Planum temporale and Heschl gyrus volume reduction in schizophrenia: A magnetic resonance imaging study of first-episode patients. *Archives of General Psychiatry, 57*(7), 692–699.

Hoffman, R. E., & Hampson, M. (2012). Functional connectivity studies of patients with auditory verbal hallucinations. *Front. Hum. Neurosci, 6*(6).

Hoftman, G. D., Volk, D. W., Bazmi, H. H., Li, S., Sampson, A. R., & Lewis, D. A. (2015). Altered cortical expression of GABA-related genes in schizophrenia: Illness progression vs developmental disturbance. *Schizophrenia Bulletin, 41*(1), 180–191.

Insel, T. R. (2010). Rethinking schizophrenia. *Nature, 468*(7321), 187–193.

Jacobi, W. U., & Winkler, H. (1928). Encephalographische studien an schizophrenen. *European Archives of Psychiatry and Clinical Neuroscience,84*(1), 208-226.

Javitt, D. C., Steinschneider, M., Schroeder, C. E., & Arezzo, J. C. (1996). Role of cortical N-methyl-D-aspartate receptors in auditory sensory memory and mismatch negativity generation: Implications for schizophrenia. *Proceedings of the National Academy of Sciences, 93*(21), 11962–11967.

Johnstone, E., Frith, C. D., Crow, T. J., Husband, J., & Kreel, L. (1976). Cerebral ventricular size and cognitive impairment in chronic schizophrenia. *The Lancet, 308*(7992), 924–926.

Kasai, K., Shenton, M. E., Salisbury, D. F., Hirayasu, Y., Onitsuka, T., Spencer, M. H., et al. (2003). Progressive decrease of left Heschl gyrus and planum temporale gray matter volume in first-episode schizophrenia: A longitudinal magnetic resonance imaging study. *Archives of General Psychiatry, 60*(8), 766–775.

Lencer, R., Bishop, J. R., Harris, M. S., Reilly, J. L., Patel, S., Kittles, R., et al. (2014). Association of variants in DRD2 and GRM3 with motor and cognitive function in first-episode psychosis. *European Archives of Psychiatry and Clinical Neuroscience, 264*(4), 345–355.

Leweke, F. M., Giuffrida, A., Wurster, U., Emrich, H. M., & Piomelli, D. (1999). Elevated endogenous cannabinoids in schizophrenia. *Neuroreport, 10*(8), 1665–1669.

Lewis, D. A., Curley, A. A., Glausier, J. R., & Volk, D. W. (2012). Cortical parvalbumin interneurons and cognitive dysfunction in schizophrenia. *Trends in Neurosciences, 35*(1), 57–67.

Lewis, D. A., Cho, R. Y., Carter, C. S., Eklund, K., Forster, S., Kelly, M. A., et al. (2008). Subunit-selective modulation of GABA type A receptor neurotransmission and cognition in schizophrenia. *The American Journal of Psychiatry, 165*(12), 1585–1593.

Lewis, D. A., Cruz, D. A., Melchitzky, D. S., & Pierri, J. N. (2001). Lamina-specific deficits in parvalbumin-immunoreactive varicosities in the prefrontal cortex of subjects with schizophrenia: Evidence for fewer projections from the thalamus. *American Journal of Psychiatry, 158*(9):1411–22.

Liddle, P. F. (1987). The symptoms of chronic schizophrenia. A re-examination of the positive-negative dichotomy. *The British Journal of Psychiatry, 151*(2), 145–151.

Lisman, J. E., Coyle, J. T., Green, R. W., Javitt, D. C., Benes, F. M., Heckers, S., et al. (2008). Circuit-based framework for understanding neurotransmitter and risk gene interactions in schizophrenia. *Trends in Neurosciences, 31*(5), 234–242.

Lupica, C. R. (1995). Delta and mu enkephalins inhibit spontaneous GABA-mediated IPSCs via a cyclic AMP-independent mechanism in the rat hippocampus. *The Journal of Neuroscience, 15*(1), 737–749.

Meador-Woodruff, J. H., Clinton, S. M., Beneyto, M., & McCullumsmith, R. E. (2003). Molecular abnormalities of the glutamate synapse in the thalamus in schizophrenia. *Annals of the New York Academy of Sciences, 1003*(1), 75–93.

Morris, H. M., Hashimoto, T., & Lewis, D. A. (2008). Alterations in somatostatin mRNA expression in the dorsolateral prefrontal cortex of subjects with schizophrenia or schizoaffective disorder. *Cerebral Cortex, 18*(7), 1575–1587.

Nakamura, M., Salisbury, D. F., Hirayasu, Y., Bouix, S., Pohl, K. M., Yoshida, T., et al. (2007). Neocortical gray matter volume in first-episode schizophrenia and first-episode affective psychosis: A cross-sectional and longitudinal MRI study. *Biological Psychiatry, 62*, 773–783.

Olney, J. W., & Farber, N. B. (1995). Glutamate receptor dysfunction and schizophrenia. *Archives of general psychiatry, 52*(12), 998-1007.

Plum, F. (1972). Prospects for research on schizophrenia. 3. Neurophysiology. Neuropathological findings. *Neurosciences Research Program Bulletin, 10*, 384–388.

Rajkowska, G., Selemon, L. D., & Goldman-Rakic, P. S. (1998). Neuronal and glial somal size in the prefrontal cortex: A postmortem morphometric study of schizophrenia and Huntington disease. *Archives of General Psychiatry, 55*(3), 215–224.

Ross, C. A., & Pearlson, G. D. (1996). Schizophrenia, the heteromodal association neocortex and development: Potential for a neurogenetic approach. *Trends in Neurosciences, 19*(5), 171–176.

Salisbury, D. F., Kuroki, N., Kasai, K., Shenton, M. E., & McCarley, R. W. (2007). Progressive and interrelated functional and structural evidence of post-onset brain reduction in schizophrenia. *Archives of General Psychiatry, 64*(5), 521–529.

Salisbury, D. F., Shenton, M. E., Griggs, C. B., Bonner-Jackson, A., & McCarley, R. W. (2002). Mismatch negativity in chronic schizophrenia and first-episode schizophrenia. *Archives of General Psychiatry, 59*(8), 686–694.

Salisbury, D. F., Shenton, M. E., & McCarley, R. W. (1999). P300 topography differs in schizophrenia and manic psychosis. *Biological Psychiatry, 45*(1), 98–106.

Salisbury, D. F., Shenton, M. E., Sherwood, A. R., Fischer, I. A., Yurgelun-Todd, D. A., Tohen, M., et al. (1998). First-episode schizophrenic psychosis differs from first-episode affective psychosis and controls in P300 amplitude over left temporal lobe. *Archives of General Psychiatry, 55*(2), 173–180.

Shenton, M. E., Dickey, C. C., Frumin, M., & McCarley, R. W. (2001). A review of MRI findings in schizophrenia. *Schizophrenia Research, 49*(1), 1–52.

Simpson, E. H., Kellendonk, C., & Kandel, E. (2010). A possible role for the striatum in the pathogenesis of the cognitive symptoms of schizophrenia. *Neuron, 65*(5), 585–596.

Smith, R. C., Calderon, M., Ravichandran, G. K., Largen, J., Vroulis, G., Shvartsburd, A., et al. (1984). Nuclear magnetic resonance in schizophrenia: A preliminary study. *Psychiatry Research, 12*(2), 137–147.

Sohal, V. S., Zhang, F., Yizhar, O., & Deisseroth, K. (2009). Parvalbumin neurons and gamma rhythms enhance cortical circuit performance. *Nature, 459*(7247), 698–702.

Tatard-Leitman, V. M., Jutzeler, C. R., Suh, J., Saunders, J. A., Billingslea, E. N., Morita, S., et al. (2015). Pyramidal cell selective ablation of N-methyl-D-aspartate receptor 1 causes increase in cellular and network excitability. *Biological Psychiatry, 77*(6), 556–568.

Thompson, P. M., Vidal, C., Giedd, J. N., Gochman, P., Blumenthal, J., Nicolson, R., et al. (2001). Mapping adolescent brain change reveals dynamic wave of accelerated gray matter loss in very early-onset schizophrenia. *Proceedings of the National Academy of Sciences, 98*(20), 11650–11655.

Thune, J. J., Uylings, H. B., & Pakkenberg, B. (2001). No deficit in total number of neurons in the prefrontal cortex in schizophrenics. *Journal of Psychiatric Research, 35*(1), 15–21.

Umbricht, D., Schmid, L., Koller, R., Vollenweider, F. X., Hell, D., & Javitt, D. C. (2000). Ketamine-induced deficits in auditory and visual context-dependent processing in healthy volunteers: Implications for models of cognitive deficits in schizophrenia. *Archives of General Psychiatry, 57*(12), 1139–1147.

van Tricht, M. J., Nieman, D. H., Koelman, J. H., van der Meer, J. N., Bour, L. J., de Haan, L., et al. (2010). Reduced parietal P300 amplitude is associated with an increased risk for a first psychotic episode. *Biological Psychiatry, 68*(7), 642–648.

Van Haren, N. E., Cahn, W., Pol, H. H., & Kahn, R. S. (2012). The course of brain abnormalities in schizophrenia: can we slow the progression?. *Journal of Psychopharmacology, 26*(5 suppl), 8-14.

Vesterager, L., Christensen, T. Ø., Olsen, B. B., Krarup, G., Melau, M., Forchhammer, H. B., et al. (2012). Cognitive and clinical predictors of functional capacity in patients with first episode schizophrenia. *Schizophrenia Research, 141*(2), 251–256.

Volk, D. W., Pierri, J. N., Fritschy, J. M., Auh, S., Sampson, A. R., & Lewis, D. A. (2002). Reciprocal alterations in pre- and postsynaptic inhibitory markers at chandelier cell inputs to pyramidal neurons in schizophrenia. *Cerebral Cortex, 12*(10), 1063–1070.

Volk, D. W., Radchenkova, P. V., Walker, E. M., Sengupta, E. J., & Lewis, D. A. (2012). Cortical opioid markers in schizophrenia and across postnatal development. *Cerebral Cortex, 22*(5), 1215–1223.

Somatic Treatments
for Psychotic Disorders

**Justin C. Ellison, Jason B. Rosenstock,
and Michael J. Marcsisin**

Introduction

Psychotic disorders, as we have seen, are biologically based, psychosocially influenced illnesses that cause significant functional effects in the lives of those who suffer from them. These are chronic illnesses, triggered by abnormal neural networks, which affect cognition, behavior, and thought, with complications that range from medical comorbidity to addiction to suicide.

Fortunately, treatments exist that can help. Although there is no cure for schizophrenia, we can provide therapies that can alleviate symptoms to the point that patients can pursue functional life goals of their choosing, achieving a quality of life that has come to be designated as "recovery"—stability, wellness, connection, peace.

In this chapter, we will focus on somatic treatments—biologically based or operationalized therapies ranging from medication to neuromodulation. These treatments play a cornerstone role in improving the lives of individuals with psychotic disorders, and we will review their mechanisms of action, risks, and appropriate use. In the next chapter, we will explore psychosocial treatments, which also play a key role in management.

Principles of Care

Somatic treatments fit into two broad philosophies of care for managing psychosis: the disease management, or chronic care model; and the biopsychosocial model. To understand how these treatments are best used, we need to appreciate these two models.

The principles of disease management draw from the chronic care models in general medicine. A century ago, physicians managed mostly acute illnesses, especially infectious, where there was a cure (at least potentially) that would eliminate the illness. Over the past few decades, medicine has shifted towards managing more chronic illnesses, like arthritis, diabetes, or hypertension, and other disorders for which there is no cure—just ways to manage the symptoms to allow people to function better. Similarly, for most psychotic disorders, disease management is the best way to conceptualize care. While we may be able to help "cure" an acute or brief psychotic disorder, conditions like schizoaffective disorder and delusional disorder tend to be chronic, and therapies focus on symptom remission rather than on complete reversal of the illness, which may not be possible anyway. Individuals who have any of these psychotic disorders will always be at risk of having future episodes of illness; treatment can help prevent relapse and alleviate symptoms when they come.

Providers should focus, then, on quality of life and functioning as much as possible, using treatments that allow individuals to heal, and to manage the illness over its various stages (from prodrome, to acute illness, to continuation and maintenance phases). Disease management supports a continuum of care, incorporating services to assist with this recovery of functioning, allowing people to reintegrate into society in roles of their choosing.

The second treatment philosophy emphasizes the importance of biopsychosocial care. Widely accepted throughout medicine, the biopsychosocial model grew out of the work of Adolf Meyer a century ago and was revived by George Engel in the 1970s. Simply put, the model encourages practitioners to think about biological, psychological, and social factors in the development and treatment of medical illness. In psychosis, this model encourages us to pursue broad, multidisciplinary treatments that can help in different ways, for a range of symptoms and issues, aided by a variety of provider types. One evidence-based example is the role of antipsychotic medication, long a mainstay of treatment. We know that medication is essential for treatment and recovery, but we also know that it is insufficient. Patients who receive only antipsychotics simply do not do as well as those who receive medication combined with psychosocial treatments: the broader approach helps to better treat symptoms and protect against relapse, improving functioning and quality of life. Physicians in solo practice generally cannot manage patients with psychotic disorders on their own; therapists, rehabilitation counselors, housing specialists, forensic service coordinators, social workers, occupational therapists, neuropsychologists, and other providers all have a role to play in improving outcomes.

Role of Somatic Therapies: An Overview

Medications are still required for the treatment of psychosis, which is important to emphasize. Many illnesses in psychiatry get better with time (e.g., conversion disorder), or respond better to psychotherapy than to medication (e.g., personality disorders). In psychotic disorders, however, there is a low placebo response, and good evidence supports the role of pharmacotherapy in treatment as superior to psychotherapy alone (American Psychiatric Association, 2004). Pharmacotherapy is particularly useful for relapse prevention; following a psychotic episode, perhaps 70% of untreated patients will relapse within nine months, versus only 30% of patients treated with antipsychotics.

These statistics should not be interpreted to mean that every patient requires maintenance or lifelong treatment. At least 10% of patients following a first episode of schizophrenia will never have another episode, and they do not require ongoing pharmacotherapy. Guidelines generally recommend one year of treatment following a first episode of illness, and if a person is symptom-free and doing well, and is thought to be a low relapse risk, consideration should be given to a taper-off medication. After a second episode, however, the relapse risk off medication is much higher, so several years of stability would be recommended before considering a trial tapering.

Although there are many antipsychotics available, several generalizations can be made about their use:

- Antipsychotics have similar efficacy, with a 60–70% response rate in acute psychosis.
- Clozapine is the "gold standard" in treatment-refractory conditions and has been demonstrated to be superior to other antipsychotics in treatment-resistant schizophrenia.
- Most antipsychotics have long half-lives (close to 24 hours), which allow for once-daily dosing.
- Antipsychotics are better at treating positive symptoms and are not as good at targeting negative or cognitive symptoms.
- Antipsychotics have significant toxicity and can lead to pronounced extrapyramidal or metabolic side effects, which limit their acceptability and require close patient monitoring.
- Non-adherence to treatment is a major issue, partly related to poor medication tolerability, partly due to other factors (cost, lack of insight, stigma, etc.).

- Newer antipsychotics ("second generation"), while having some tolerability benefits, are no more effective than older medications (Sikich et al., 2008; Jones et al., 2006) and are significantly more expensive (in fact, they are generally much more expensive than any other psychotropics).
- There are limited data on combinations of antipsychotics, or augmentation strategies, and cost and tolerability issues make such practices suspect.
- Aggressive side-effect management is important to assuring adherence and quality of life.

We will explore these points in more detail as we review the specific drug classes and their use, including polypharmacy/augmentation, side-effect management, and uses across illnesses stages and in special populations.

In addition, we will discuss the role of non-pharmacological somatic therapies, which absolutely have a place in the care of patients with psychotic disorders. Electroconvulsive therapy (ECT), in fact, predates pharmaceuticals, and was developed in the in 1930s specifically for the treatment of schizophrenia. Although more used now for mood disorders, ECT remains an effective management option for many patients with schizophrenia. And newer "neuromodulation" interventions like repetitive transcranial magnetic stimulation (rTMS) and transcranial direct-current stimulation (tDCS) may carve out a niche in the armamentarium to treat psychotic disorders, although their proper and effective use is less clear at this point.

Pharmacotherapy: Brief Background on Development and Use

The beginnings of the modern-day pharmacotherapy for schizophrenia came about serendipitously with an observation by Henri Laborit, a Parisian surgeon. At the time, chlorpromazine was administered as a preoperative anesthetic, and Laborit noted its strong tranquilizing effects and subsequent reduction in preoperative anxiety. In 1952, Delay and Deniker, on the basis of these findings, administered chlorpromazine to institutionalized patients experiencing psychotic symptoms, with noted reductions in hallucinations, delusions, and agitation. This successful clinical intervention led to the widespread use of chlorpromazine in psychotic patients, which in turn sparked the development of a class of medications with dopamine (specifically D2) receptor blockade as the primary mechanism of therapeutic efficacy for schizophrenia.

Dopamine-receptor blocking agents were initially termed *neuroleptics* (loosely translated as "to seize the neuron," from the Greek *leptikos,* "to seize") due to the belief that the drug-induced Parkinsonism associated with their use was crucial to attaining efficacy. The use of the term "neuroleptic" to describe this class of medications is no longer appropriate, as it focused on non-therapeutic side effects; therefore, calling these medications "antipsychotics" has become standard nomenclature.

The main therapeutic action of antipsychotics centers on the dopamine (DA) hypothesis of schizophrenia. This theory conceptualizes the positive symptoms of schizophrenia as resulting from excess DA in the mesolimbic tract of the central nervous system (CNS). This is in line with the model of drug-induced symptoms of psychosis demonstrated with amphetamines, cocaine, and L-dopa. However, the DA hypothesis may fail to capture the pathophysiology behind the negative and cognitive symptoms of schizophrenia.

The introduction of clozapine in the United States in the 1990s ignited the second wave of antipsychotic development. Clozapine demonstrated that an agent could be effective in managing symptoms of psychosis with minimal to no extrapyramidal symptoms (EPS). A unique second generation of antipsychotic medications with high serotonin (5HT2A) receptor antagonism in relation to D2 antagonism was developed based on this new prototypical agent.

Table 6.1 Clinical Effects of Receptor Antagonism by Antipsychotics

Receptor	Clinical Effect of Antagonism
Dopamine (D2)	Mesolimbic pathway (basal ganglia)—treatment of positive symptoms
	Nigrostriatal pathway (substantia nigra)—EPS
	Tuberoinfundibular pathway (hypothalamus)—increased prolactin
	Mesocortical pathway (prefrontal cortex)—secondary negative symptoms
Serotonin (5HT2A)	Treatment of positive symptoms; may increase dopamine release in prefrontal cortex and reduce phasic mesolimbic dopamine output
Serotonin (5HT2c)	Weight gain
Muscarinic (μ1)	Anticholinergic effects (xerostomia, constipation, blurred vision, hot dry skin, confusion), sedation
Histamine (H1)	Increased appetite, sedation
Alpha (α1)	Orthostatic hypotension

Common terms used to delineate the two current classes of antipsychotics are *typical* versus *atypical*. "Atypicality" refers to the newer agents' lower rates of EPS. However, the classes differ in a variety of other ways, so these terms are not adequately descriptive. Generally, the two classes are called *first-generation antipsychotics* (FGAs) and *second-generation antipsychotics* (SGAs), and they will be referred to as such for consistency throughout this chapter. FGAs and SGAs antagonize several receptor subtypes to different degrees. Clinical effects of this antagonism are outlined in Table 6.1.

Pharmacotherapy: Clinical Treatment Guidelines and Antipsychotic Efficacy

Multiple organizations have published clinical guidelines on the treatment of schizophrenia. It is important to bear in mind that the sources of information utilized to compile the recommendations in each guideline may vary in terms of strength of supporting evidence. For example, the Patient Outcomes Research Team on Schizophrenia (PORT) sets a threshold of evidence of at least two randomized controlled trials to put forth a treatment recommendation (Buchanan et al., 2009). The Texas Medication Algorithm Project for Schizophrenia, on the other hand, will utilize expert opinion or consensus to provide recommendations on areas not as well studied, including clozapine non-response and antipsychotic combination therapy (Moore et al., 2007). These guidelines can provide, as their names suggest, "guidance" on treatment decisions, but they should not be wholly relied upon in deciding the appropriate course of treatment. As always, the management of schizophrenia should be individualized and patient-centric.

The comparative effectiveness of various antipsychotic medications was examined in a landmark clinical trial, the Clinical Antipsychotic Trials of Intervention Effectiveness (CATIE), sponsored by the National Institute of Mental Health (NIMH) in 2005. The CATIE trial randomized participants to treatment with olanzapine ($n = 330$), risperidone ($n = 333$), quetiapine ($n = 329$), ziprasidone ($n = 183$), and the mid-potency FGA, perphenazine ($n = 257$). The primary outcome was "time to all-cause discontinuation" (i.e., discontinuation secondary to lack of efficacy or intolerable side effects). By the 18-month study endpoint, 74% of patients discontinued treatment. Patients randomized to treatment with olanzapine discontinued treatment significantly less frequently (64%) than the other agents. However, the primary reason cited for discontinuation of olanzapine was more frequently weight gain or metabolic symptoms versus other groups. Extrapyramidal symptoms (EPS) were cited as the main cause for discontinuation in the perphenazine group. The time to discontinuation for intolerable side effects did not differ significantly between treatment groups. There were no significant differences in efficacy rating scales between the FGA perphenazine and the SGAs (Lieberman et al., 2005; Stroup et al., 2006; McEvoy et al., 2006).

A meta-analysis conducted by Leucht and colleagues (2009) examined 150 randomized, double-blind studies comparing SGAs and FGAs on the basis of overall efficacy, positive and negative symptoms, depression, relapse, quality of life, EPS, weight gain, and sedation. Four SGAs outperformed FGAs on overall efficacy, with small to moderate effect sizes (clozapine −0.52, olanzapine −0.28, risperidone −0.13, and amisulpride −0.31). The other five SGAs (aripiprazole, sertindole, quetiapine, ziprasidone, and zotepine) were no more efficacious than FGAs for positive or negative symptoms, and all agents induced side effects to varying degrees. This evidence supports weighing efficacy, side-effect profile, and treatment cost to formulate an individualized treatment plan.

Figure 6.1 depicts a consolidated portrayal of the most current medication treatment guidelines for schizophrenia available.

First-Generation Antipsychotics

FGAs (Table 6.2, Table 6.3) are believed to exert their clinical effects through antagonism of postsynaptic D2 receptors in the mesolimbic and to a certain extent in the mesocortical areas of

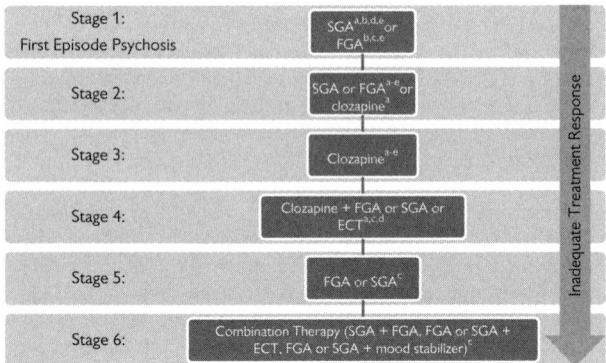

Stage 1: First Episode Psychosis	SGA[a,b,d,e] or FGA[b,c,e]
Stage 2:	SGA or FGA[a,e] or clozapine[a]
Stage 3:	Clozapine[a,e]
Stage 4:	Clozapine + FGA or SGA or ECT[a,c,d]
Stage 5:	FGA or SGA[c]
Stage 6:	Combination Therapy (SGA + FGA, FGA or SGA + ECT, FGA or SGA + mood stabilizer)[c]

Inadequate Treatment Response

Figure 6.1 Summary of current treatment guidelines on schizophrenia.
[a] American Psychiatric Association (APA, 2004)
[b] Patient Outcomes Research Team (PORT, 2009)
[c] Texas Medication Algorithm Project (TMAP, 2007)
[d] International Psychopharmacology Algorithm Project (IPAP, 2005)
[e] National Institute for Health and Care Excellence (NICE—UK, 2014)

Table 6.2 First-Generation Antipsychotics

Medication Name (Generic/Brand);Potency/ Chlp Eq*;Class	Dosage Forms	Adult Dosing Schedules	Dose Adjustments
Haloperidol/Haldol® High/2 Butyrophenone	*Tablet:* 0.5, 1, 2, 5, 10, 20 mg *Oral solution:* 2 mg/ml *Injectable (immediate-release):* 5 mg/ml *Injectable (long-acting):* 50, 100 mg/ml	*Initiate 0.5–5 mg BID or TID (depending on symptom severity)* *Usual range:* 5–40 mg	*Renal:* No specific recommendations *Hepatic:* No specific recommendations
Fluphenazine/Prolixin® High/2 Phenothiazine	*Tablet:* 1, 2.5, 5, 10 *Oral elixir:* 2.5 mg/mL *Oral solution:* 5 mg/mL *Injectable (immediate-release):* 2.5 mg/mL *Injectable (long-acting):* 25 mg/mL	*Initiate:* 2.5–10 mg q 6–8 hours *Usual range:* 1–40 mg/day	*Renal:* Use with caution (non-dialyzable) *Hepatic:* Use with caution

(continued)

Table 6.2 Continued

Medication Name (Generic/Brand);Potency/ Chlp Eq*;Class	Dosage Forms	Adult Dosing Schedules	Dose Adjustments
Pimozide/Orap® High/2 Diphenylbutyl-piperidine	*Tablet:* 1, 2 mg	*Initiate:* 2 mg/day and titrate to clinical response *Usual range:* 2–10 mg/day	*Renal:* No specific recommendations *Hepatic:* Consider dose reduction in severe hepatic insufficiency
Thiothixene/Navane® High/4 Thioxanthene	*Capsule:* 1, 2, 5, 10 mg	*Initial:* 6–10 mg daily (divided doses) *Usual range:* 5–60 mg/day	*Renal:* Use with caution (non-dialyzable) *Hepatic:* Consider dose reduction
Trifluoperazine/ Stelazine® High/5 Phenothiazine	*Tablet:* 1, 2, 5, 10 mg	*Initial:* 2–5 mg BID *Usual range:* 15–20 mg/day	*Renal:* Use with caution (non-dialyzable) *Hepatic:* Consider dose reduction

Perphenazine/Trilafon® Mid/8–10 Phenothiazine	*Tablet:* 2, 4, 8, 16 mg	*Initial:* 4–8 mg TID *Usual range:* 8–64 mg/day	*Renal:* No specific recommendations *Hepatic:* Consider dose reduction
Loxapine/Loxitane® Mid/10 Dibenzoxazepine	*Capsule:* 5, 10, 25, 50 mg *Inhalation powder:* 10 mg	*Initial:* 10 mg BID *Usual range:* 20–250 mg/day (PO)	*Renal:* No specific recommendations *Hepatic:* No specific recommendations
Chlorpromazine/Thorazine® Low/100 Phenothiazine	*Tablet:* 10, 25, 50, 100, 200 mg *Injection (immediate-release):* 25 mg/mL	*Initial:* 100–200 mg/day in divided doses; increase 20–50 mg/day q3–4 days as indicated	*Renal:* No specific recommendations *Hepatic:* Consider dose reduction

*Chlp Eq = chlorpromazine equivalents (i.e., the respective dose in milligrams equivalent to 100 mg chlorpromazine).

BID, twice daily; TID, thrice daily

Table 6.3 Cytochrome P450 Enzyme Interactions with First-Generation Antipsychotics

Medication	Metabolic Pathway	Clinically Significant Drug Interactions
Chlorpromazine	CYP 2D6 (major), CYP 1A2 (minor), CYP 3A4 (minor)	Propranolol[5], QTc-prolonging agents (e.g., thioridazine, pimozide, ziprasidone)[7], tamoxifen[5,6]
Fluphenazine	CYP 2D6 (major)	Strong CYP 2D6 inhibitors (e.g., paroxetine, fluoxetine, bupropion, quinidine)[2]
Haloperidol	CYP 2D6 (major), CYP 3A4 (major), CYP 1A2 (minor)	Nilotinib[1,6]
Loxapine	CYP 1A2, CYP 2D6, CYP 3A4	Metoclopramide[7], CNS depressants[3]
Perphenazine	CYP 2D6	Ziprasidone
Pimozide	CYP 3A4 (major), CYP 1A2 (minor)	Fluvoxamine[6], clarithromycin[2,6], ketoconazole[6], QTc-prolonging agents[7]
Thioridazine	CYP 2D6 (major), CYP 2C19 (minor)	CYP 2D6 inhibitors[2], QTc-prolonging agents[6]
Thiothixene	CYP 1A2 (major)	Thioridazine[6]
Trifluoperazine	CYP 1A2 (major)	Fluvoxamine[2], ciprofloxacin[2]

[1] May require increase in antipsychotic dose
[2] May require decrease in antipsychotic dose
[3] Combination requires increased monitoring
[4] Concomitant agent may require dose increase
[5] Concomitant agent may require dose decrease
[6] Avoid combination when possible
[7] Combination is contraindicated

the CNS. Evidence supports that the FGAs are all equally efficacious in reducing the core positive symptoms of schizophrenia
when given in equivalent doses. However, their side-effect profiles vary based upon their potency at the D2 receptor (low-,
mid-, and high-potency) (Figure 6.2). The low-potency agents
(chlorpromazine, thioridazine) have a high affinity for alpha-
adrenergic, histaminergic, and muscarinic receptors, which gives
them a higher risk of anticholinergic, sedative, and hypotensive
effects. High-potency agents (haloperidol, fluphenazine, thiothixene, trifluoperazine) are more likely to cause acute extrapyramidal symptoms, tardive dyskinesia and dystonia, and prolactin
elevation, but they have a much lower incidence of anticholinergic effects and orthostasis. Mid-potency agents (molindone,
loxapine, perphenazine), as their name implies, are in the middle
of the pack in terms of acute and chronic EPS, sedation, anticholinergic effects, and hypotension.

Several FGAs deserve specific attention in order to better
understand the pharmacology and side effects of the most commonly used agents.

Haloperidol
Haloperidol, a butyrophenone derivative, is structurally unrelated to the phenothiazines (fluphenazine, thiothixene, etc.),

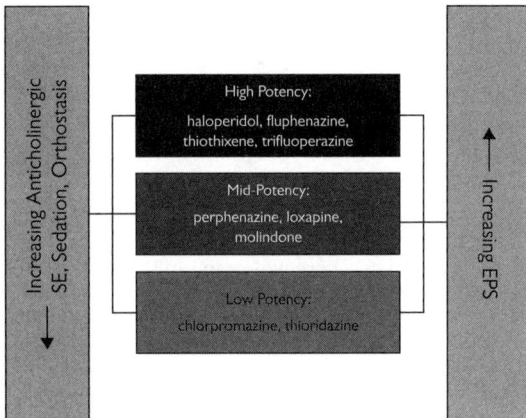

Figure 6.2 Relative side effects associated with high-, mid-, and
low-potency FGAs.

but it has a similar pharmacodynamic and side-effect profile. It is considered a high-potency D2 antagonist and as such is associated with a higher risk of EPS-related side effects. Its low affinity for alpha receptors allows it to be titrated rapidly in acutely psychotic or agitated patients without concern for orthostatic hypotension or falls. The primary pathway of its metabolism is through CYP2D6 and 3A4, with CYP1A2 playing a minor role. Haloperidol tablets have a bioavailability that is 40–80% of parenteral dosage forms. Therefore, an equivalent oral dose will be approximately 1.5 times that of the intramuscular (IM) or intravenous (IV) formulation.

There is a decanoate ester long-acting injectable (LAI) formulation of haloperidol available. Conversion to the LAI formulation can be achieved either by administering 10 times the oral dose the patient is stabilized on, or by administering 20 times the oral dose for a loading-dose regimen. The loading dose will result in reaching therapeutic serum levels of haloperidol more rapidly and allow the discontinuation of the oral medication after completion of the loading regimen. The usual conversion, without a load, will require that the oral dose be continued for at least one month prior to being gradually tapered (McEvoy, 2006). Injections require the "Z-track technique" to prevent loss of medication, abscesses, or subdermal lumps. This technique can be more painful than standard injections and involves stretching the skin to one side over the injection site, injecting the medication slowly into the muscle, and then waiting 10 seconds prior to removing the needle. The injections should preferably be rotated among six sites to prevent subdermal scarring, and the maximum injection volume should be limited to three milliliters (mL).

Fluphenazine

Fluphenazine, a piperazine phenothiazine, is a commonly utilized high-potency FGA. It undergoes hepatic metabolism mediated primarily by CYP2D6. There is also an LAI decanoate ester formulation of fluphenazine available. Unlike haloperidol decanoate, the LAI formulation of fluphenazine is released relatively quickly, with a time of maximum concentration (Tmax) of approximately 24 hours. Therefore, the oral medication can be decreased by 50% upon administration of the first injection and discontinued after the second. The oral-to-decanoate conversion most commonly utilized is 1.25 times the oral dose given every 2–4 weeks. For example, a patient stabilized on fluphenazine 10 mg orally would be converted to 12.5 mg of fluphenazine decanoate given every two weeks. A double-blind study conducted by Carpenter and colleagues (1999) reported no difference in relapse, symptoms, or side effects between patients stabilized on either an every two weeks or every six weeks injection interval. This demonstrates that longer dosing intervals without risk of relapse may be an option if dose reduction is indicated. The "Z-track technique" must also be used with fluphenazine decanoate to ensure delivery of the full volume of medication.

Perphenazine

Perphenazine is a mid-potency phenothiazine. It has a half-life of approximately 9–12 hours once reaching steady-state plasma concentrations after 72 hours. Metabolism of perphenazine is moderated through CYP2D6. Caution should be taken when it is administered with potent CYP2D6 inhibitors due to increased risk of side effects, such as EPS, resulting from increased perphenazine concentrations. Perphenazine was selected as the FGA comparator utilized in the landmark CATIE trial due to its moderate risk for motoric and metabolic side effects versus the high- and low-potency FGAs, respectively. It still sees use in clinical practice because of its more "balanced" side-effect profile and low risk for metabolic complications compared to other FGAs and SGAs.

Chlorpromazine

Chlorpromazine is a low-potency aliphatic phenothiazine. It is rarely utilized for the treatment of psychotic disorders these days because of potent alpha-adrenergic, muscarinic, and histaminergic blockade and associated side effects. Chlorpromazine also has a dose-dependent risk of QTc prolongation, similar to the structurally related agent thioridazine. Baseline and periodic electrocardiogram monitoring should accompany its use.

The oral bioavailability of chlorpromazine is poor, and its absorption is highly impacted by the presence of food or concomitant therapy with medications such as antacids. Chlorpromazine induces its own metabolism, which will cause a 25–33% decrease in serum levels after one to three weeks of treatment. Additionally, it is a major substrate of CYP2D6, so the presence of concomitant strong inhibitors will affect its clearance. Plasma levels following IM injections will be 4–10 times higher than those achieved through administration of the same oral dose.

Second-Generation Antipsychotics

The pharmacological profiles of the SGAs (Table 6.4, Table 6.5) differ from those of the FGAs in four main ways, as their activity can include:

1. potent serotonin (5HT) receptor blockade in addition to dopamine (D2) blockade,
2. D2 partial agonism and subsequent stabilization of dopamine neurotransmission (aripiprazole),
3. partial agonism of 5HT1A (aripiprazole, clozapine, quetiapine, ziprasidone),
4. rapid dissociation and looser binding to the D2 receptor.

In general, the SGAs have a lower risk for EPS than the FGAs; however, they do carry a higher cardiometabolic risk. The risk of weight gain (>7% body weight) for the SGAs is ranked as follows: clozapine = olanzapine ≥ quetiapine > risperidone = paliperidone > iloperidone > lurasidone = asenapine = ziprasidone = aripiprazole (American Diabetes Association et al., 2004). A meta-analysis of 48 head-to-head randomized controlled trials found that olanzapine produced more weight gain than other SGAs and equal weight gain to clozapine. Olanzapine also produced higher cholesterol elevations than aripiprazole, risperidone, and ziprasidone, but no difference compared to clozapine or quetiapine. Quetiapine was shown to cause greater cholesterol elevations than risperidone and ziprasidone. Lastly, glucose elevations were higher for olanzapine than for aripiprazole, quetiapine, risperidone, and ziprasidone, with no difference compared to clozapine (Rummel-Kluge et al., 2010).

The weight gain and metabolic side effects related to SGAs necessitate the monitoring recommendations outlined later in this chapter. Annual incidence rates of tardive dyskinesia (TD) for the SGAs are estimated at 0.5–1.5%, versus 4–5% for FGAs. 5HT2A-receptor antagonism has been demonstrated to facilitate tonic dopamine release in the mesocortical and nigrostriatal pathways, helping to prevent EPS and cognitive blunting associated with strong D2 blockade (Meltzer et al., 2003). The D2 receptor occupancy of SGAs is greatly outweighed by 5HT2A occupancy at lower dosages.

The elimination half-lives of the SGAs range from 18–103 hours once steady-state plasma concentrations are reached in three to five half-lives, with the exception of ziprasidone and quetiapine. This enables SGAs to be converted to once-daily dosing after tolerability has been established. Although the

Table 6.4 Second-Generation Antipsychotics

Medication Name (Generic/Brand)	Dosage Forms	Adult Dosing Schedules	Dose Adjustments
Aripiprazole/Abilify®	*Tablet:* 2, 5, 10, 15, 20, 30 mg *ODT:* 10, 15 mg *Injectable (short-acting):* 9.75 mg/1.3 mL *Injectable (long-acting):* 300 mg/vial and 400 mg/vial *Solution:* 1 mg/mL	*Initial:* 10–15 mg/day, titrate at 2-week intervals *Usual range:* 15–40 mg	*Renal/Hepatic:* No dose adjustment necessary
Asenapine/Saphris®	*Sublingual tablet:* 5, 10 mg	*Initial:* 5 mg BID (no benefit demonstrated with higher doses)	*Renal/Hepatic:* No dose adjustments necessary; use not recommended in severe hepatic impairment

(continued)

Table 6.4 Continued

Medication Name (Generic/Brand)	Dosage Forms	Adult Dosing Schedules	Dose Adjustments
Clozapine/Clozaril®	*Tablet:* 12.5, 25, 50, 100, 200 mg *ODT:* 12.5, 25, 100 mg	*Initial:* 12.5–25 mg/day, titrate by 25–50 mg/day to target of 300–450 mg/day *Usual range:* 350–600 mg	*Renal/Hepatic:* No specific recommendations
Iloperidone/Fanapt®	*Tablet:* 1, 2, 4, 6, 8, 10, 12 mg	*Initial:* 1 mg BID, increase by 2 mg/day to target dose of 12–24 mg/day	*Renal:* No adjustments necessary *Hepatic:* Use not recommended

Lurasidone/Latuda®	Tablet: 20, 40, 80, 120 mg	Initial: 40 mg daily taken with food Usual range: 40–160 mg/day	Renal: Initial dose of 20 mg/day and max of 80 mg/day in moderate—severe impairment Hepatic: Initial dose of 20 mg/day and max of 80 mg/day in moderate impairment and max of 40 mg in severe impairment
Olanzapine/Zyprexa®	Tablet: 2.5, 5, 7.5, 10, 15, 20 mg ODT: 5, 10, 15, 20 mg Injection (short-acting): 10 mg/vial (5 mg/ml after reconstitution) Injection (long-acting): 210, 300, 405 mg/vial	Initial: 2.5–10 mg/day Usual range: 20–40 mg/day	Renal: Initial dose of 5 mg/day should be considered Hepatic: Childs Pugh Class A and B, no adjustment necessary

(continued)

Table 6.4 Continued

Medication Name (Generic/Brand)	Dosage Forms	Adult Dosing Schedules	Dose Adjustments
Paliperidone/Invega®	*Tablet (ER):* 1.5, 3, 6, 9 mg *Injectable (long-acting):* 39, 78, 117, 156, 234 mg prefilled syringes	*Initial:* 6 mg/day; increases should not exceed 3 mg every 5 days *Usual range:* 9–12 mg	*Renal:* CrCl 50–79 ml/min: initiate at 3 mg, max 6 mg/day CrCl 10–49 ml/min: initiate at 1.5 mg, max 3 mg/day CrCl <10 ml/min: use not recommended *Hepatic:* Child-Pugh Class A and B no adjustment required

Quetiapine/ Seroquel®	*Tablet (IR):* 25, 50, 100, 200, 300, 400 mg *Tablet (ER):* 50, 150, 200, 300, 400 mg	*Initial (IR):* 25 mg BID; titrate in 25–50 mg increments, given 2–3 times daily, to a target range of 300–400 mg/ day by day 4 *Usual range (IR):* 300–750 mg/day *Initial (ER):* 300 mg/day; *Usual range (ER):* 400–800 mg/day	*Renal:* No specific recommendations *Hepatic:* Initiate IR tablets at 25 mg/day and increase by 25–50 mg increments/ day; initiate ER tablets at 50 mg/day and increase by 50 mg/day increments
Risperidone/ Risperdal®	*Tablet:* 0.25, 0.5, 1, 2, 3, 4 mg *ODT:* 0.5, 1, 2, 3, 4 *Solution:* 1 mg/mL *Injectable (long-acting):* 12.5, 25, 37.5, 50 mg	*Initial:* 1–2 mg/day *Usual range:* 4–8 mg/day	*Renal/Hepatic:* Recommend initial dose of 0.5 mg BID; may increase dose 0.5 mg BID; increases above 1.5 mg BID should be completed over 1 week intervals

(continued)

Table 6.4 Continued

Medication Name (Generic/Brand)	Dosage Forms	Adult Dosing Schedules	Dose Adjustments
Ziprasidone/Geodon®	*Capsule:* 20, 40, 60, 80 mg *Injectable (short-acting):* 20 mg/mL	*Initial:* 20 mg BID with food; dose adjustments at ≥48 hour intervals	*Renal:* No adj. necessary in mild-mod. impairment - Use IM with caution (cyclodextrin sodium excipient) *Hepatic:* No adj. necessary in mild-mod. impairment

ODT = orally disintegrating tablet; IR = immediate release; ER = extended release; CrCl = Creatinine Clearance

Table 6.5 Cytochrome P450 Enzyme Interactions with Second-Generation Antipsychotics

Medication	Metabolic Pathway	Clinically Significant Drug Interactions
Aripiprazole	CYP 2D6, 3A4	CYP 3A4 inducers (e.g., carbamazepine, phenobarbital, phenytoin, rifamycin)[1], strong CYP 3A4 inhibitors (e.g.,.. ketoconazole, clarithromycin, verapamil)[2], strong CYP 2D6 inhibitors (e.g., paroxetine, fluoxetine, bupropion, quinidine)[2]
Asenapine	Glucuronidation by UGT1A4 and CYP 1A2	Strong CYP 1A2 inhibitors (e.g., fluvoxamine, ciprofloxacin, and primaquine)[2], paroxetine[2,6]
Clozapine	CYP 1A2 (major), 3A4, 2D6, 2C19 (minor)	Strong CYP 1A2 inhibitors[2], CYP 1A2 inducers[1], CYP 3A4 inducers[1], polycyclic aromatic hydrocarbons (cigarette smoke)[1], CNS depressants (e.g., benzodiazepines, alcohol)[6]
Iloperidone	CYP 2D6 and CYP 3A4 (major)	CYP 2D6 inhibitors[2], CYP 3A4 inhibitors[2]
Lurasidone	CYP 3A4	Strong CYP 3A4 inhibitors or inducers[7], moderate CYP 3A4 inhibitors[2]
Olanzapine	CYP 1A2 (major), CYP 3A4 (minor) and glucuronidation	CYP 1A2 inducers[1], CNS depressants[6], antihypertensives[5]

Table 6.5 Continued

Medication	Metabolic Pathway	Clinically Significant Drug Interactions
Paliperidone	Primarily renal elimination	QTc-prolonging agents[3]
Quetiapine	CYP 3A4 (major) and CYP 2D6 (minor)	CNS depressants[3,6], antihypertensives[3], CYP 3A4 inducers[1], CYP 3A4 inhibitors[2],
Risperidone	CYP2D6 (major) and CYP 3A4 (minor)	Moderate–strong CYP 2D6 inhibitors[2], antihypertensives[5]
Ziprasidone	Aldehyde oxidase (major) CYP 3A4 and CYP 1A2 (minor)	Carbamazepine[1], ketoconazole[2], QTc-prolonging agents[7]

[1] May require increase in antipsychotic dose
[2] May require decrease in antipsychotic dose
[3] Combination requires increased monitoring
[4] Concomitant agent may require dose increase
[5] Concomitant agent may require dose decrease
[6] Avoid combination when possible
[7] Combination is contraindicated

pharmacokinetic profile of agents such as clozapine would suggest the need for more frequent dosing, the actual duration of action is significantly longer. This discrepancy is partly due to the variation between receptor kinetics in the periphery versus that of the CNS. Most antipsychotics are highly lipophilic and are thus eliminated slowly from lipid-rich areas, such as the CNS. For example, a pharmacokinetic study utilizing positron emission tomography (PET) demonstrated a significant variation between the mean single-dose plasma half-lives of risperidone and olanzapine (24.2 and 10.3 hours) and the time until 50% reduction in the striatal D2 receptor occupancy of either agent was observed (75.2 and 66.6 hours, respectively) (Tauscher & Jones, 2002). Consolidation to a single daily dosing regimen results in lower pill burden and enhanced patient adherence.

The SGAs that have recently come to market have not demonstrated a significant improvement in efficacy over previous antipsychotics. More importantly, they may not be covered or may be non-preferred by some insurance plans and have a high out-of-pocket cost for the patient. High cost of treatment greatly limits the clinical use of the newer SGAs (e.g., lurasidone, iloperidone, and asenapine) in the treatment of psychosis. If treatment with a newer SGA is clinically appropriate, it is important to determine if the medication is covered by insurance and check with the patient's pharmacy or insurance carrier to determine if a prior authorization is needed. This will avoid any interruptions in treatment if the patient brings in the prescription to be filled and finds they cannot afford the medication or they have to wait for prior authorization before the medication can be filled.

Let us next examine several specific SGAs, to better understand the pharmacology and side effects of the most commonly used agents.

Risperidone/Paliperidone (Risperdal®, Invega®)

Risperidone is a benzioxazole derivative with antagonist activity at dopamine (D1-4), serotonin (5-HT1A, 2A, 2C), alpha-adrenergic (α1,2), and histamine (H1) receptors. Paliperidone, or 9-hydroxyrisperidone, is the active metabolite of risperidone, formed by oxidative metabolism through CYP2D6. The pharmacological profile of risperidone is more prototypical of the SGAs at the lower end of the dosage range (2–5 mg) with potent 5HT2A antagonism in relation to its D2 antagonism. However, further titration to dosages above 6 mg pushes the D2 receptor occupancy to approximately 77%. The additional D2 antagonism

at higher doses of risperidone results in a pharmacological profile more closely resembling the FGAs and their higher propensity for EPS. Risperidone and paliperidone have the highest risk
of hyperprolactinemia of the SGAs, due to extensive D2 blockade in the tuberoinfundibular dopamine pathway. The anterior
pituitary, responsible for the release of prolactin, sits outside
blood–brain barrier. The higher D2 binding affinity and concentration of paliperidone at this site gives it a slightly higher risk of
hyperprolactinemia than risperidone. The clinical sequelae that
may result from excess prolactin production include amenorrhea
in females, and sexual dysfunction, galactorrhea, gynecomastia,
and bone mineral density changes in both males and females.
However, prolactin levels do not acutely correlate with these
adverse events and are only of concern in actively symptomatic
patients. Risperidone also has a moderate risk of cardiometabolic concerns and weight gain.

Paliperidone is available as a sustained-release oral formulation that utilizes osmotic pressure to slowly push the active
compound out of a laser-drilled pore in an insoluble tablet. This
causes it to reach its Tmax in 24 hours versus the more rapid
1–1.5-hour absorption and higher peak concentration (Cmax)
of risperidone. The faster absorption and higher Cmax give risperidone more concentration-dependent side effects, such as
orthostasis and excess sedation, versus paliperidone. Therefore,
risperidone is routinely dosed twice daily when first initiated,
then consolidated to once-daily dosing once tolerability is established. Paliperidone should be dosed once daily in the morning
due to the kinetics of its sustained-release dosage formulation.
The patient should be counseled that a "ghost shell" of the insoluble tablet may be present in stool and can cause complications
if the patient has any gastrointestinal narrowing or obstruction.

Both risperidone and paliperidone are available in long-acting
injectable dosage forms. The long-acting injectable formulation of risperidone (Risperdal Consta®) is available as 12.5, 25,
37.5, and 50 mg intramuscular injections administered every
two weeks. The risperidone is suspended in glycolic acid-lactate
copolymer microspheres that are slowly hydrolyzed, resulting
in a delayed absorption of approximately three weeks. This
delay in release necessitates a three-week overlap of oral risperidone when newly initiating a patient on the LAI formulation.
Paliperidone, on the other hand, has a palmitate formulation that
can be dosed monthly (39, 79, 117, 156, and 234 mg) and does

not require an oral overlap after the initial loading dose of 234 mg given in the deltoid on day 1, followed by a 156 mg deltoid injection on day 8. The dose of paliperidone palmitate needs to be reduced to 156 mg day 1 followed by 117 mg day 8 (both administered in the deltoid) in patients with mild renal impairment (creatinine clearance $\geq$ 50 mL/min to < 80 mL/min). Both injections should still be administered in the deltoid and followed by a monthly maintenance dose of 78 mg given in either the deltoid or gluteal muscle. Paliperidone palmitate should not be administered in patients with severe renal impairment (creatinine clearance below 50 mL/min).

Risperidone is primarily metabolized through CYP2D6, which is important to note because this particular hepatic isoenzyme is prone to extensive genetic polymorphisms distributed based upon racial demographics. CYP2D6 activity is very low to absent in 5–8% of Caucasians and 2–5% of African-Americans and Asians due to this variability in genetic expression. In patients who express this decreased activity enzymatic phenotype, the half-lives of risperidone and 9-hydroxyrisperidone will be approximately 17 hours and 30 hours, respectively. The addition of a potent CYP2D6 inhibitor would also increase the total exposure, known as the area under the curve (AUC), for risperidone and place the patient at higher risk for adverse side effects. Paliperidone is primarily excreted unchanged (57%) in the urine and does not undergo hepatic metabolism.

Ziprasidone (Geodon®)

Ziprasidone is a benzisothiazolyl piperazine derivative with very potent antagonist activity at the 5HT2A receptor in relation to its D2 antagonist activity. It also has antagonist activity at the 5HT1C, 5HT1D, and 5HT2C receptors, moderate affinity for α1, and low affinity for H1. Both clozapine and ziprasidone share 5HT1A agonist activity; however, ziprasidone is the only SGA to exhibit serotonin and norepinephrine reuptake inhibition. This would in theory suggest antidepressant actions, but there is little evidence to support this. Ziprasidone is one of the few SGAs to require twice-daily dosing. Food will increase the absorption of ziprasidone by two-fold; therefore, it must also be administered with a meal of at least 500 calories. Ziprasidone is also available as a rapid-acting IM injection FDA-indicated (US Food and Drug Administration) for use in acute agitation in adults.

Ziprasidone has a lower propensity to cause weight gain, dyslipidemia, increased fasting triglycerides, or insulin resistance.

However, ziprasidone does carry the greatest risk for QTc prolongation of the SGAs. The Pfizer 054 study demonstrated QTc prolongation as a class effect for SGAs. Ziprasidone was observed to extend the QTc interval by a mean of 15.9 msec, whereas thioridazine extended the QTc by a mean of 30.1 msec. Other antipsychotics included in the Pfizer study (olanzapine, quetiapine, risperidone, haloperidol) demonstrated a mean QTc interval increase of 1.7–7.1 msec (Harrigan & Miceli, 2004). To add context, the mean diurnal variation in QTc is approximately 75 msec for a given individual. No cases of *torsades de pointes* were observed in the 4,571 ziprasidone-treated patients. Clinically, this necessitates caution and careful consideration of the risks and benefits when contemplating the initiation of, or continued treatment with, ziprasidone. Use should be avoided in patients with underlying cardiac issues, electrolyte abnormalities (hypokalemia or hypomagnesaemia), congenital long-QT syndrome, or those co-medicated with agents affecting cardiac function (particularly antiarrhythmics of class Ia—disopyramide, procainamide, quinidine; and class III—amiodarone, dofetilide, sotalol).

Ziprasidone is largely metabolized through aldehyde oxidase, accounting for two-thirds of its breakdown, with CYP3A4 and CYP1A2 playing only a minor role. When administered concomitantly, carbamazepine induction of CYP3A4 has the potential to decrease the plasma concentration of ziprasidone by 36%. Alternatively, co-administered ketoconazole can increase the AUC and Cmax of ziprasidone by 33% and 34%, respectively, through CYP3A4 inhibition.

Asenapine (Saphris®)

The chemical structure of asenapine closely resembles that of the tetracyclic antidepressant mirtazapine. Both agents share alpha2, 5HT2A, 5HT2C and H1 antagonism. However, asenapine has additional D2 antagonism as well as activity at other serotonin receptor subtypes, including partial 5HT1A agonism and 5HT7 antagonism. Asenapine is metabolized by glucuronidation through UGT1A4 and CYP1A2. Strong CYP1A2 inhibitors, such as fluvoxamine and ciprofloxacin, may raise the serum levels of asenapine, increasing the risk of concentration-dependent side effects.

The bioavailability of asenapine is severely limited by extensive first-pass metabolism. The sublingual formulation of asenapine bypasses this effect and results in a Tmax of approximately

0.5–1.5 hours. The time of onset is not as rapid as might be expected due to compartmentalization in the oral mucosa. Upon administration, the compound is rapidly dissolved in the saliva and transported into the mucosal membranes until a pseudo-equilibrium is reached. The oral cavity has a limited surface area, which results in the remainder of the solid compound's being swallowed and rendered inactive before a true equilibrium can be achieved. The limited surface area available for absorption requires split-day dosing for doses greater than 5 mg even though asenapine has a 24-hour half-life. The rate-limiting step in the absorption of asenapine is the transfer from the mucosal membranes into systemic circulation.

Iloperidone (Fanapt®)

Iloperidone, a benzisoxazole derivative, is a newer SGA with high 5HT2a antagonism in relation to D2 antagonist activity. However, it is differentiated by its potent alpha1 blockade, which results in high rates of orthostasis and sedation. This limits how rapidly it can be titrated and usually necessitates splitting the dose when it is being initiated, even though its 18–33-hour half-life should allow for daily dosing. The remainder of the pharmacological profile of iloperidone is rounded out by moderate alpha2, 5HT1b/d, and 5HTt7 antagonism, and partial 5HT1a agonism. This agent has low incidence of dyslipidemias but carries a moderate risk for weight gain. There were no changes in serum glucose with iloperidone in the registry trials. However, a dose-dependent increase in QTc prolongation was reported.

Iloperidone is primarily metabolized through CYP2D6 and CYP3A4. The addition of a potent inhibitor of either enzyme has the potential to increase the serum concentration of iloperidone; therefore, it is recommended to decrease the dose of iloperidone by 50% if concomitant administration is deemed necessary.

Quetiapine (Seroquel®)

Quetiapine is a dibenzothiazepine derivative structurally related to clozapine. It is available in both an immediate release (IR) as well as an extended release (XR) formulation. Quetiapine has the lowest D2 blockade of the SGAs, which confers a low risk of EPS and hyperprolactinemia. Its low risk of EPS makes quetiapine particularly useful in the subset of patients with Parkinson's disease or Lewy body dementia requiring treatment with an antipsychotic. The high H1 and α1 blockade results in the high incidence of sedation, dizziness, and orthostasis observed with quetiapine. The active metabolite of quetiapine, norquetiapine, possesses some differing pharmacological activity than the parent compound. These include inhibition at the norepinephrine transporter (NET), 5HT2c, 5HT7, and α2A receptors, in addition to partial 5HT1a agonism. The XR formulation of quetiapine may be associated with lower incidence of peak concentration-dependent side effects (e.g., sedation); however, its cost and non-superior efficacy to the IR formulation limits its clinical use. Both formulations have a similar, intermediate risk for diabetes, dyslipidemias, weight gain, and QTc prolongation.

The mean terminal half-life of quetiapine is approximately six hours, allowing it to reach steady-state concentrations within two days of administration. Quetiapine IR is rapidly absorbed upon administration and will reach peak concentrations within 1.5 hours post-dose. Alternatively, the XR formulation will reach its Cmax six hours post-dose. The delay in onset of the XR formulation makes the IR more beneficial for patients experiencing difficulties with sleep latency in addition to symptoms of psychosis. Administration of quetiapine XR with a high-fat meal, approximately 800–1000 calories, can cause clinically relevant increases in its Cmax and AUC (44–52 and 20–22%, respectively). These administration effects are not observed with the IR formulation. It is recommended that the XR formulation be administered on an empty stomach or with a light meal, if necessary.

Quetiapine undergoes extensive hepatic metabolism. In vitro data support CYP3A4 as the main hepatic isoenzyme involved in the metabolism of quetiapine to both its major active N-desalkyl metabolite (norquetiapine) and its major inactive sulfoxide metabolite. In cases of hepatic insufficiency, the oral clearance may be reduced by up to 30% and the AUC increased three-fold, possibly requiring dose adjustment. No similar dose adjustments are suggested in renal insufficiency. If administration of concurrent potent CYP3A4 inhibitors (e.g., ketoconazole, itraconazole, ritonavir) or inducers (e.g., phenytoin, carbamazepine, rifampin) is necessary, dose adjustment of quetiapine will be necessary to avoid increased or decreased exposure, respectively. Quetiapine has no clinically significant impact on the pharmacokinetics of other medications. However, quetiapine may have additive sedative and hypotensive effects when combined with similar agents or alcohol.

Olanzapine (Zyprexa®)

Olanzapine is a thienobenzodiazepine structurally similar to clozapine, though with more potent D2 and 5HT2a antagonism. It also has high affinity for 5HT2c, H1, and α1 receptors and moderate affinity for M1-5 and 5HT3 receptors. Olanzapine reaches its Cmax approximately six hours post-dose. After one week of administration, olanzapine will reach steady-state concentrations and have an elimination half-life of 30 hours. Olanzapine, similar to clozapine, has one of the highest risks of the SGAs for causing cardiometabolic side effects and significant weight gain.

Olanzapine undergoes extensive first-pass metabolism through direct glucuronidation and oxidation mediated primarily by CYP1A2. Only 60% of the parent compound will reach systemic circulation following oral administration. A reduction in olanzapine serum levels and exposure is observed with concurrent administration of potent CYP1A2 inducers (e.g., rifampin, phenytoin, and carbamazepine). The polyaromatic hydrocarbons in cigarette and cannabis smoke can also appreciably induce CYP1A2. At 8–10 cigarettes (about a half pack daily), CYP1A2 induction will be saturated, resulting in an increase in olanzapine clearance by approximately 50%. Should smoking cessation occur, the resultant reversal in enzymatic induction will cause an increase in olanzapine serum levels. Therefore, changes in patient smoking status should be consistently monitored, and adjustments to the olanzapine dose should be made accordingly. This interaction should be kept in mind when patients are being admitted and discharged from smoke-free facilities. Potent inhibitors of CYP1A2 (e.g., fluvoxamine) will decrease the clearance of olanzapine.

In addition to the oral capsule formulation, olanzapine is also available as an orally disintegrating tablet, a short-acting injectable, and a long-acting injectable formulation. Due to concerns about excessive orthostatic hypotension, the short-acting injectable should be dosed at least two hours after the initial 10 mg IM dose or four hours after a second 10 mg IM dose. It should also be separated from IM doses of benzodiazepines by at least 60 minutes due to similar concerns about orthostasis and excessive CNS depression. The safety of doses of olanzapine IM in excess of 30 mg in a 24-hour period (10 mg given every 2–4 hours) has not been studied clinically. The patient should be assessed for orthostatic hypotension and subsequent doses be withheld if significant orthostasis or syncope is observed.

There is a risk evaluation and mitigation strategy (REMS) in place due to the 0.2% risk of post-injection delirium/sedation syndrome (PDSS) associated with the LAI formulation of olanzapine (Relprevv®). PDSS is caused by supratherapeutic levels of olanzapine resulting from accidental intravascular placement of the injection. The turbidity in the bloodstream leads to the rapid dissolution of olanzapine pamoate. The injection must be given in a facility with readily available access to emergency response services, and the patient must be continuously observed for three hours post-injection by a healthcare professional for symptoms consistent with olanzapine overdose. The majority of observed cases of PDSS occurred with this three-hour window; however, there have been reports of the event occurring outside of the three-hour observation period. This risk is present with each injection administration, and a history of tolerability does not confer a lower risk for PDSS with future injections. The high administrative burden of coordinating the post-injection monitoring limits its use in routine clinical practice.

Aripiprazole (Abilify®)
Aripiprazole, a quinolone derivative, has a unique pharmacology that includes partial agonist activity at the D2 and 5HT1a receptors in addition to antagonist activity at the 5HT2a receptor. Partial D2 agonism results in lower rates of EPS and may help alleviate hyperprolactinemia caused by other agents with more potent D2 antagonism, such as risperidone or haloperidol. The partial D2 agonism may also cause nausea and vomiting early in treatment and be somewhat activating in certain patients. In this subset of patients, morning dosing will help avoid disrupting sleep architecture. Aripiprazole is also differentiated by its lack of M1 and H1 activity and low risk of inducing weight gain, fasting triglyceride elevations, or insulin resistance. However, this does not mean it cannot induce weight gain in select individuals, particularly in the child and adolescent population. The 75-hour elimination half-life of aripiprazole may be of particular benefit in patients who have difficulty with medication adherence.

Aripiprazole is metabolized by dehydrogenation and hydroxylation catalyzed by CYP3A4 and CYP2D6 and N-dealkylation through CYP3A4. Concurrent administration of the strong CYP3A4 inhibitor ketoconazole with aripiprazole was demonstrated to increase the AUC of the parent compound by 63%

and its active metabolite (dehydro-aripiprazole) by 77%. When aripiprazole is administered with strong CYP3A4 inhibitors, its dose should be reduced by 50%. Strong CYP2D6 inhibitors demonstrate a similar effect on the AUC of aripiprazole, but reduce its metabolism to dehydro-aripiprazole. Administration of quinidine with aripiprazole resulted in an increase in the AUC of aripiprazole of 112% and a decrease in the AUC of dehydro-aripiprazole by 35%. When initiating a potent CYP2D6 inhibitor, such as paroxetine or fluoxetine, in a patient stabilized on aripiprazole, the dose of aripiprazole should be decreased by 50%. If either a potent CYP3A4 or CYP2D6 inhibitor were to be withdrawn, a similar dose increase of aripiprazole would be needed to address the reversal of enzymatic inhibition. Potent inducers of CYP3A4, such as carbamazepine, will have the opposite effect. If concurrent administration is clinically indicated, the dose of aripiprazole should be doubled.

Similar precautions need to be considered in those considered to be poor CYP2D6 metabolizers. This phenotype is expressed in approximately 8% of Caucasians and 3–8% of African Americans and results in an 80% increase in the AUC of aripiprazole and 30% decrease in dehydro-aripiprazole AUC compared to the general population. The resultant net exposure will be approximately 60% higher. Therefore, aripiprazole should be initiated at half the normal dosage in known CYP2D6 poor metabolizers. Aripiprazole is unlikely to exert any clinically relevant pharmacokinetic effect on other agents metabolized through cytochrome P450.

An orally disintegrating tablet, short-acting IM injection, liquid, and long-acting injection are all available. The short-acting IM injection has a bioavailability of 100% versus the 87% of the oral tablet. Therefore, the Cmax and AUC within two hours of administration will be greater for the injection; however, the overall 24-hour exposure to aripiprazole from both dosage forms will be comparable. The tablet, orally disintegrating tablet, and liquid formulation can be substituted at a 1:1 ratio. The LAI formulation should only be given by gluteal injection. The normal starting dose for most patients will be 400 mg IM monthly. However, the aforementioned dose adjustments for the oral formulation are also necessary when administering the LAI formulation of aripiprazole concomitantly with strong CYP3A4 or CYP2D6 inhibitors or inducers for longer than 14 days or in poor CYP2D6 metabolizers (see Table 6.6).

Table 6.6 Long-Acting Injectable (LAI) Antipsychotics

Medication	PO to LAI Conversion	Dosage	Dosing Interval	Loading Dose Available	PO Overlap
Fluphenazine decanoate	10 mg PO = 12.5 mg Q3 weeks IM	*Initial:* 12.5–25 mg *Target:* 12.5–50 mg	Q2-4W	No; Insufficient evidence	Decrease PO by 50% after first injection; d/c PO after second injection
Haloperidol decanoate	10–20 × PO dose	10–15 × PO dose administered monthly; 100 mg maximum for first injection if haloperidol dec. naïve; balance may be given in 3–7 days if > 100 mg	Q4W	Yes; 20 × PO dose first injection then 10 × PO dose maintenance	Continue PO x 2–3 injections if loading dose not used
Aripiprazole monohydrate (Abilify Maintena®)	400 mg IM Q month	*Initial:* 400 mg IM monthly; 300 mg IM monthly (poor CYP2D6 metabolizers, concomitant strong CYP2D6 or 3A4 inhibitors, or side effects at higher dose) 200 mg monthly (poor CYP2D6 metabolizers taking CYP3A4 inhibitors, concomitant strong CYP2D6 and 3A4 inhibitors)	Q month	No	Continue PO x 14 days

	PO dose	IM dose first 8 weeks	IM dose maintenance				
Olanzapine pamoate **(Zyprexa Relprevv®)**	10 mg/day	210 mg Q2W or 405 mg Q4W	150 mg Q2W or 300 mg Q4W	*Initial:* 150–300 mg IM Q2W or 405 mg Q 4W	Yes	Q2W or Q4W	Not required
	15 mg/day	300 mg Q2W	210 mg Q2W or 405 mg Q4W	*Target:* 300 mg Q2W or 405 mg Q4W			
	20 mg/day	300 mg Q2W	300 mg Q2W				
Paliperidone palmitate (Invega Sustenna®)	**PO dose**	Initiate with 234 mg IM on day 1 and 156 mg IM on day 8 (both deltoid). *Mild renal impairment (CrCl ≥50 mL/min and < 80mL/min):* Initiate with 156 mg IM on day 1, then 117 mg IM day 8.		**IM dose**	Yes	Q4W	Not required
	3 mg/day			39–78 mg			
	6 mg/day			117 mg			
	12 mg/day			234 mg			
	Mild renal impairment			78 mg			
Risperidone long-acting injection (Risperdal Consta®)	**PO dose**	**IM dose**		*Initial:* 25 mg IM Q2W with PO overlap x 3W	No	Q2W	Continue PO x 3 weeks
	2–3 mg	25 mg		*Target:* 25–50 mg IM Q2W			
	4–5 mg	37.5 mg					
	6 mg	50 mg					

Q = every; W = week[s]; PO = oral; IM = intramuscular; CrCl = creatinine clearance

Lurasidone (Latuda®)

Lurasidone is a benzisothiazol derivative with high affinity for D2, 5HT2a, and 5HT7 receptors, moderate affinity for 5HT1a and α2c receptors, and little to no affinity for M1 and H1 receptors. Its pharmacological action is attributed to antagonist activity at all of the aforementioned receptor subtypes, aside from partial agonist activity at 5HT1a. Like that of aripiprazole and ziprasidone, the metabolic profile of lurasidone is relatively clean, with low risk for weight gain or dyslipidemias. The absorption of lurasidone, like ziprasidone, is greatly increased by administration in a fed versus fasted state. Taking lurasidone with a 350-calorie meal will increase its AUC and Cmax by two and three times, respectively. This effect was seen independently of the dietary fat content of the meal, and drug exposure did not increase any further when the size of the meal was greater than 350 calories. Lurasidone has an elimination half-life of approximately 18 hours and will reach steady-state concentration at a given dose within seven days of consistent administration.

The primary pathway of metabolism for lurasidone is via oxidative N-dealkylation, hydroxylation of norbornane ring, and S-oxidation catalyzed by CYP3A4. Lurasidone was not observed to have any appreciable effects on the metabolism or concentrations of other medications. However, since it is a major substrate of CYP3A4, concurrent administration of strong inhibitors (e.g., fluconazole) and strong inducers (e.g., rifampin) is contraindicated. The dose of lurasidone should not exceed 40 mg daily if concurrent administration of a moderate CYP3A4 inhibitor (e.g., diltiazem) is necessary. The recommended total daily dose should also not exceed 40 mg in patients with moderate to severe renal or hepatic impairment.

Clozapine (Clozaril®)

Clozapine, a tricyclic dibenzodiazepine, was the prototypical agent that shifted the focus of antipsychotic development towards agents with higher 5HT2A affinity relative to D2. It has a unique and complex pharmacology that consists of high affinity and antagonist activity at 5HT2A, 5HT2C, 5HT3, 5HT7, H1, α1A,2A, M1,3, D1-5, and agonist activity at M4. Clozapine undergoes extensive hepatic metabolism primarily via CYP1A2. CYP2D6, CYP3A4, and CYP2C19 are involved to a lesser extent. N-desmethyl clozapine (NDMC), also called norclozapine, is the primary active metabolite of clozapine. Clozapine-n-oxide, the other main metabolite of clozapine, is mostly inactive.

The effect of clozapine on this array of receptor subtypes, both centrally and in the periphery, is responsible for its extensive side-effect profile. These side effects range from the more common and bothersome sialorrhea, constipation, orthostatic hypotension, and sedation, to the rare yet more serious seizures, myocarditis, cardiomyopathy, and agranulocytosis. A dose-dependent risk for seizure was described by Devinsky and colleagues (1991) in a retrospective review of premarketing data for 1,418 clozapine-treated patients. At doses less than 300 mg, the risk is 1%: at doses from 300–600 mg, the risk is 2.7%; and at doses greater than 600 mg, the associated risk is 4.4%. Evidence for increased risk of seizures at higher serum clozapine levels is limited to case reports of tonic-clonic seizures occurring at serum levels above 1300 ng/mL. Agranulocytosis is a rare side effect, occurring in slightly less than 1% of clozapine-treated patients. It was first identified in a population of Finnish patients in 1975, eight cases of which were fatal. In response, clozapine did not come on the U.S. market until its superior efficacy in treatment-refractory schizophrenia was demonstrated by a randomized controlled trial conducted by Kane and colleagues in 1988. Clozapine was then approved for use in patients with schizophrenia who have failed to respond to adequate trials of other antipsychotics. The superior efficacy of clozapine in treatment-refractory schizophrenia versus other antipsychotics is supported by multiple randomized controlled trials, including phase II of the CATIE trial (Leucht et al., 2009; McEvoy et al., 2006). Due to concerns about agranulocytosis, however, the patient, prescriber, and dispensing pharmacy must all be registered with the FDA's clozapine risk-evaluation and mitigation strategy (REMS) program prior to dispensing clozapine. The clozapine REMS program is mandated by the FDA to track absolute neutrophil count (ANC) values and ensure that patients who have experienced agranulocytosis while on clozapine are not rechallenged. ANC values reported to the REMS program must be above 1500/μL, or 1000/μL in patients with benign ethnic neutropenia (BEN), in order to safely begin treatment with clozapine. Clozapine monitoring may be increased in frequency or treatment discontinued if the ANC falls below these values during the course of treatment.

It is also important to keep in mind the cholinergic rebound that may occur with abrupt discontinuation of clozapine (e.g., in the case of agranulocytosis). This withdrawal is more severe than with other SGAs due to the potent muscarinic antagonism of clozapine. The patient should be monitored for profuse sweating, headache, nausea, vomiting, and diarrhea. There is some evidence for initiating an anticholinergic medication, such as benztropine, for a short time to counteract these withdrawal effects.

Clozapine and norclozapine serum levels can be clinically useful. We know, for instance, that patients are more likely to respond to clozapine when the level is above 350 ng/mL. There is no consensus or consistent evidence to support an upper limit of therapeutic efficacy, but at higher levels, the increasing side-effect burden begins to outweigh the marginal benefit gained by raising the dose. Once a patient has responded to a stable dose of clozapine, drawing a serum level can provide a useful basis for comparison if levels are drawn in the future. Other indications for obtaining serum levels include:

1. *CNS toxicity* (which can result from elevated serum levels)
2. *Drug–drug interactions* (especially following the addition or withdrawal of agents that can appreciably affect CYP1A2 or CYP3A4 metabolic pathways)
3. *Smoking status changes* (e.g., a patient stops or starts smoking, which can affect clozapine metabolism as well)
4. *Non-adherence concerns* (e.g., breakthrough symptoms occur despite steady dosing)

Polypharmacy

As we have seen, antipsychotics, saddled with safety issues and efficacy gaps, may have limited utility for many patients with psychosis. In the CATIE trial, for instance, three-quarters of patients taking antipsychotics for schizophrenia ended up switching to a different medication by the end of 18 months, with switches being due either to lack of efficacy or to intolerability (Lieberman et al., 2005). Many individuals require more aggressive somatic treatment, including the addition of other medications to augment a primary antipsychotic as a way of helping it work better.

Unfortunately, very little evidence exists about appropriate strategies for augmentation. We know that up to 20% of patients with primary psychotic disorders end up taking more than one antipsychotic medication (particularly young male patients who have high symptom burdens), but there is little evidence that such antipsychotic polypharmacy actually improves outcomes.

It definitely increases costs and produces more side effects for patients. As such, there have been many efforts to limit such antipsychotic polypharmacy unless clearly warranted.

Probably the best-studied antipsychotic polypharmacy approach is "clozapine plus": prescribing a second antipsychotic to a treatment-refractory patient already taking clozapine. When such patients have partial responses, providers often feel extremely limited, not wanting to take a patient off of the gold standard treatment. Additionally, there are theoretical reasons to combine a strong D2-blocking agent (e.g., an FGA) with clozapine, which binds more weakly to D2. There are about 10 trials, for instance, of adding risperidone, which has strong D2-binding, but unfortunately few showed added benefit. There are also trials of aripiprazole and FGAs like amisulpride (not available in the United States), most of which have demonstrated added efficacy.

There has been more attention given to combining other psychotropics with antipsychotics to augment response, particularly for specific target symptoms like depression, aggression, or negative symptoms. The classic augmentation strategy for antipsychotics is adding lithium, although the evidence supporting this is surprisingly limited. Other mood stabilizers have been studied as add-ons, with good data supporting the use of valproate as a way to accelerate response to acute psychosis, and lamotrigine has been shown to be effective as a clozapine augmenter. Beta-blockers and benzodiazepines may help for aggression or anxiety in the context of psychosis, and antidepressants may help with depressive or negative symptoms. Newer studies have looked at amino acids like glycine or serine, or fish oil, as antipsychotic augmenters, and early data look promising.

When facing very sick patients with overwhelmed families, desperate to "do something" that might help, and with insurance companies demanding "active treatment" to justify ongoing care, providers may experience intense pressure to add medications to existing antipsychotics. However, given the limited data, the strategy for treatment-refractory patients should generally follow established clinical care guidelines. Sequential monotherapies of antipsychotics should be trialed, each at a good dose and duration, until response. Clozapine should be used as the gold standard for refractory patients, and augmentation should be trialed only for specific comorbid symptoms or for clozapine partial response.

Side-Effect Management

As we have seen, antipsychotics carry a significant burden of toxicity, which can interfere with adherence and cause significant distress, morbidity, and even mortality for patients who use these medications. Because of these risks, we need to be particularly careful in monitoring for and aggressively managing emergent side effects in patients taking antipsychotics. Let us more closely examine how we might manage side effects like EPS (including tardive dyskinesia [TD]), metabolic syndrome, and other problems related to antihistamine, anticholinergic, or antiadrenergic medication effects. We will specifically address clozapine and some of the risks of that medication, as well as their management strategies.

Extrapyramidal side effects include dystonia, Parkinsonism (including muscular rigidity, tremor, and gait changes), and probably related phenomena like akathisia and tardive dyskinesia. Although more likely to emerge from FGA use, EPS can be seen from any dopamine-blocking medication, whenever the nigrostriatal pathway in the basal ganglia is affected (usually at D2-receptor occupancy of 70% or above). Table 6.7 reviews the different EPS phenomena in order to help practitioners identify these side effects. Incidence estimates are "ballpark" figures based on FGA trials; EPS is of course much less likely to result from SGAs. In terms of risk, remember that, for all these forms of EPS, the most important and significant risk factor is the dose "intensity" of the antipsychotic: higher doses of high-potency D2-blockers is more likely to produce EPS, including TD, if given for longer durations. Having one form of EPS also predisposes a person to other forms.

In addition to tardive dyskinesia, patients on antipsychotics may also develop tardive dystonia or even tardive akathisia. Evidence on best management of tardive dystonia and tardive akathisia is limited, but practitioners are likely to use agents similar to what is used for acute conditions. Decrease in antipsychotic dose or a switch to clozapine should also be considered.

Although management will be the emphasis in this section, we should remember that prevention is even better. EPS can be prevented through several obvious ways:
- Start with a low-potency FGA, or an SGA.
- Limit the dose/duration of the antipsychotic.
- Avoid use in at-risk populations.
- Consider anticholinergic prophylaxis in high-risk patients.

Table 6.7 Extrapyramidal Side Effects from Antipsychotics

EPS	Acute Dystonia	Parkinsonism	Akathisia	Tardive Dyskinesia
Symptoms	Torticollis	Cogwheel rigidity	Subjective restlessness	Involuntary
	Oculogyric crisis	Masked facies	Fidgeting	Irregular
	Laryngospasm	Tremor	Pacing	Choreoathetoid
	Other tonic activity	Akinesia	Inability to sit still	Perioral
		Stooped posture		Distal→proximal
		Gait changes		
Onset (after med start)	Hours to Days [90% with 3 days]	Days to Weeks	Hours to Months [85% within 1 week]	After 3 months [May be years]
Incidence	10% [2–90%]	20% [2–90%]	25% [14–75%]	15–25% [3–4% annual risk]

(continued)

Table 6.7 Continued

EPS	AcuteDystonia	Parkinsonism	Akathisia	Tardive Dyskinesia
Risks	Younger males	Older females	Polypharmacy	Older females
	IM administration	Family history of Parkinson's or mood disorders	Mood disorders	Brain injury, seizure
	Mood disorders		Substance use	Intellectual disability
			Palliative care	Mood disorders
				Diabetes
				Smoking
Treatments	Diphenhydramine	Anticholinergics	Beta blockers	Clozapine
	Benztropine	Amantadine	Benzodiazepines	Buspirone
	[Intramuscular]		Anticholinergics	Amantadine
			Amantadine	Benzodiazepines
			Nicotine	Aripiprazole
			Mirtazapine	Mirtazapine

Anticholinergics (e.g., benztropine) can both prevent and treat EPS by restoring outflow balance in the basal ganglia; although there is a theoretical risk of worsening psychosis, in practice, this does not occur (probably because this dopamine and cholinergic balance is more important to nigrostriatal outflow rather than in the mesolimbic or mesocortical pathways). Unfortunately, anticholinergics make medication regimens more complicated, and they can cause side effects of their own (cognitive problems, constipation, blurry vision, and so on). If possible, it would be better not to have to use such agents.

Although conservative use of anticholinergics is generally recommended, if patients do develop EPS, it is important to treat it aggressively. Standard strategies for management would include lowering the dose, switching to a lower-potency FGA or an SGA, or using "antidotes" (especially anti-Parkinsonian agents—see Table 6.8) when possible. Because EPS can be so debilitating, it is important for providers to regularly screen for symptoms in the history and on exam.

Certainly these "antidotes" need to be used carefully, for several reasons. These side-effects medications have side effects of their own, as we noted, causing significant functional impairment for patients and carrying long-term risks. Importantly, not every patient needs side-effect medications for maintenance: perhaps only 10–15% require ongoing treatment, in part because patients may not require antipsychotic maintenance therapy at the same dose that caused EPS in the first place (dose reductions may obviate the need for side-effect meds). Ideally, the goal would be to try to minimize a patient's antipsychotic over time, cutting down after a few months of stability to the "minimum effective dose," which would then allow reduction or elimination of the anti-Parkinsonian medication.

The situation is a bit more complicated in tardive dyskinesia, because there is essentially no good treatment or antidote for the condition. Because of that, the emphasis should be on prevention. Fortunately, TD is not as irreversible as previously believed, but for many it is, and because it is so disfiguring and can potentially cause such significant morbidity, efforts should be made to avoid it. Partly this involves careful monitoring over time using standardized rating scales (e.g., Abnormal Involuntary Movement Scale, or AIMS) to track for symptoms every six to twelve months. At the first sign of dyskinetic movements, patients should be counselled on the implications and what their

Table 6.8 Anti-Parkinsonian Medication Options

Class [Action]	Agent	Initial Dose	Typical Dose	Max Dose	Notes
Anticholinergic [M1 Antagonist]	Benztropine	1	2	6	Abusable, cognitive problems
	Trihexyphenidyl	1	10	15	More stimulating, abusable
Dopamine Agonist	Amantadine	100	200	400	Useful in late-life, especially for akinesia; may exacerbate psychosis
Beta blocker [Noradrenergic Antagonist]	Propranolol	30	60	120	Three times daily dosing typically; use caution in reactive airway disease, monitor vital signs closely
	Atenolol	25	50	100	May have better central nervous system penetration, less sedation
Antihistamine [H1 Antagonist]	Diphenhydramine	25	50	100	Intramuscular for dystonia; sedating
Benzodiazepine [GABA Agonist]	Lorazepam	1	2	6	Effective for akathisia

options might be. Although dose reduction could trigger a rapid increase in movements due to withdrawal dyskinesia, ultimately reduction and elimination of the offending agent is likely to help reduce or eliminate the movement side effects. A switch to clozapine would be the treatment of choice for TD; if this is not possible, numerous antidotes have been tried with varying efficacy (the most promising being tetrabenazine, high-dose buspirone, branched-chain amino acids, and benzodiazepines).

EPS has long been a significant issue in patients who take antipsychotics, but with the rise of SGA-prescribing, metabolic side effects have overtaken EPS as the most significant toxicity to monitor and manage. Antipsychotics can cause weight gain, hypertension, hyperglycemia, and hyperlipidemia. The details on metabolic side effects are beyond the scope of this chapter (risks, causes, monitoring, and treatments). However, several general points can be made. Like with EPS, it is better to prevent such side effects than to try to manage them. For metabolic toxicity, prevention strategies might include:

• Choose a lower-risk agent (e.g., a weight-neutral SGA)
• Minimize dose/duration of use
• Consider prophylactic behavioral interventions (e.g., weight-loss groups)
• Consider prophylactic pharmacological interventions (e.g., metformin)

Monitoring is important, with consensus recommendations (ADA, 2004) calling for baseline checks of body mass index (BMI), waist circumference (WC), glucose, hemoglobin A1c, and lipid profile. BMI and WC should be checked essentially at every visit with the patient thereafter. Metabolic labs are drawn at three months after starting an antipsychotic and annually thereafter.

Should metabolic side effects emerge, prescribers need to have a careful risk–benefit discussion with patients and other involved physicians, to determine how best to manage the issue. Sometimes it is best or preferred to switch antipsychotics to a lower-risk agent. Lowering the dose doesn't usually help as much as stopping the agent completely. Behavioral and pharmacological interventions can help, depending on the specific metabolic issue that has arisen; such interventions might include medications like topiramate and metformin, or diet and exercise strategies given in groups or individually. Prevention and management of metabolic toxicity is particularly important, given the high morbidity and mortality associated with this class of medication, including (on average) a shorter lifespan by decades, due in part to metabolic complications.

Various other side effects besides EPS and metabolic syndrome are associated with antipsychotics, including anticholinergic (constipation, dry mouth, cognitive problems), antihistaminic (sedation), antiadrenergic (orthostasis), sexual (often linked to hyperprolactinemia), and cardiac (QTc prolongation) side effects. General strategies in addressing any of these problems would be to focus on careful monitoring, avoid the additive risk of polypharmacy, lower the medication dose, change agents, or use "antidotes." Routine labs or tests are not generally indicated in the prevention of, or screening for, these side effects, except in certain situations (e.g., electrocardiograms for patients on intravenous haloperidol in an intensive care setting, or routine orthostatic vital signs when someone is starting clozapine). Otherwise, providers can generally just screen for these during their exams and do any further work-up if needed (e.g., checking a prolactin if a patient complains of lower libido). Specific antidotes are beyond the scope of this chapter but might include stool softeners, stimulants, salt, or bromocriptine, depending on the side effect being targeted.

Finally, clozapine carries with it a high burden of side effects that must be managed, including sialorrhea, enuresis, seizure risk, and of course agranulocytosis, which could lead to death. Routine blood monitoring is required for this agent—weekly for the first six months, biweekly for the next six months, and monthly thereafter, assuming no drops in neutrophil counts below 1500. Risk for agranulocytosis is low (<1%), with most cases occurring in the first six weeks of use; beyond six months the risk becomes extremely low, but still above zero. Agranulocytosis is an idiosyncratic risk, unlike seizure risk, which is more directly dose-related: the faster the dose titration, and the higher the dose, the more likely it is that a patient will have a seizure. Therefore, dose titration should be gradual (maximum 25 mg every two days) and dosing should not exceed 900 mg/day. Constipation can be very problematic and must be aggressively managed to avoid obstruction. Drooling is annoying and can occur in 10% of clozapine patients; drooling is related to both increased salivation and decreased clearance of secretions. This side effect can be managed behaviorally (e.g., gum chewing) or pharmacologically (e.g., ipratropium, anticholinergics, or other antidotes) if dose reduction is not possible.

Management Across Stages: Prodrome, Acute, Stabilization, Maintenance

Strategies for using somatic therapies may vary, depending on the stage of psychotic illness. What a person needs in the early prodromal phase may be very different than what a more chronically ill individual requires for maintenance. Exploring these differences, along with related issues like adherence, long-acting injectables, and medication-switch strategies may help provide better disease management across the lifespan.

As we have seen in earlier chapters, the onset of psychosis may be sudden but is more likely to be insidious, with florid psychotic symptoms preceded by milder prodromal symptoms for varying lengths of time. In this prodromal phase, patients are more responsive to antipsychotics, should they be required at all, and typically lower doses can be used to good effect. There is some limited evidence that early use of antipsychotics may reduce conversion to a full disorder in high-risk patients (Mokhtari & Rajarethinam, 2013). This area is fraught with controversy because of the risks of such interventions, and the relative safety of alternative psychosocial interventions, which may be at least as effective, if not more. In addition, other medications, such as antidepressants, may be just as effective as antipsychotics at forestalling psychotic conversion, without some of the motor or metabolic side effects of antipsychotics.

Once acute or florid psychotic symptoms emerge, the treatment options become clearer, as antipsychotics are clearly indicated. Goals of treatment during this acute stage of illness include developing an alliance with the patient and their family, adequately controlling and preventing harmful behavior, reducing acute symptoms of the disorder, and facilitating a rapid return to good community functioning. Antipsychotics can help achieve these goals, along with augmenting agents as reviewed. Frequently, antipsychotics may need to be given in rapidly dissolving oral forms, or in intramuscular forms, to rapidly manage acute psychotic crises or to prevent non-adherence.

In the continuation or stabilization phase, psychotic symptoms begin to subside and recovery begins. Patients are vulnerable to relapse, and risk factors include stress, non-adherence, insomnia, substance use, and a whole host of other factors. Antipsychotic use should be continued at least for the first year after a full psychotic episode to prevent relapse, but the dosing may be lowered to avoid side effects and allow for higher levels of community functioning.

In the stable or maintenance phase, patients can remain on the minimum effective antipsychotic dose to allow for further psychosocial treatment and a full recovery. While treatment of positive symptoms tends to be emphasized in acute and stabilization phases, negative symptoms become more important in the stable phase, as they are more likely to interfere with a return to full function. In a patient with more than one psychotic episode, experts often suggest perhaps five years of continuous antipsychotic treatment with good symptom control before considering reduction or discontinuation of the medication, but this is a shared decision and needs to be made flexibly based on personal values, symptoms, and history.

Even if a patient stays on the medication, adherence remains an ongoing concern. Providers are often poor at predicting which patients are non-adherent, and perhaps 50% of patients with psychotic illness do not take medication anywhere near as often as prescribed. The use of long-acting injectable (LAI) antipsychotic medication can help prevent non-adherence, or at least make it easier to identify when patients have stopped their medication; LAIs may also be convenient and have fewer side effects, making them a good choice for maintenance treatment for many.

Should a patient require a change in antipsychotic medication during the maintenance phase, clinicians should be careful in terms of which switch strategy should be used for which patients. Although providers and patients often have much anxiety about this issue, the best evidence suggests that there is little difference among the strategies (see, for example, Weiden et al., 2014). Immediate or gradual switches, with or without cross-tapering, seem to make little difference in terms of relapse risk or adverse effects. The strategy should be individualized, with patient preference and capacity, as well as current level of symptoms, determining which strategy to choose.

Special Populations

Two populations pose specific challenges when prescribing antipsychotic medication: late-life individuals and women who are pregnant or postpartum. Although antipsychotics are still commonly used in both groups, caution must be taken to avoid toxicity.

In late life, reduced hepatic metabolism requires that prescribers cautiously dose antipsychotics, starting at lower doses, raising the dose gradually and slowly, and keeping the dose low. Effective doses may be much lower in elderly patients (e.g., chlorpromazine equivalents of 25–100, rather than the usual 300). Besides the metabolic issues, elderly individuals are more vulnerable to nervous system effects of antipsychotics; they are at increased risk of acute extrapyramidal side effects, tardive dyskinesia, and general cognitive toxicity. More recent work (e.g., Maust et al., 2015) has suggested higher mortality rates for geriatric patients taking antipsychotics, particularly FGAs like haloperidol, but perhaps with SGAs as well. However, there are mixed data about this issue, and much of it comes from the dementia literature rather than from studies with psychotic disorder subjects.

For women who are pregnant, data are limited on the safety of antipsychotics. Chlorpromazine has been the best-studied, and although some research has suggested possible increases in congenital malformations from first-trimester exposure, the bulk of studies have demonstrated no increased risk, and most observers feel that both first- and second-generation antipsychotics are probably safe (Robinson, 2012). There does not appear to be an increased risk of birth complications, for instance. Nevertheless, behavioral effects and long-term effects from early fetal exposure remain unknown, so most physicians recommend avoiding antipsychotics in the first trimester if possible. Unfortunately, it is not always possible to do so, and untreated psychosis presents a risk to the fetus and the pregnant woman. Therefore risk–benefit discussions need to take place to determine whether and how to use antipsychotics during pregnancy. If antipsychotics need to be used, it may be best to consider SGAs like quetiapine, or high-potency FGAs.

In late pregnancy, antipsychotics carry more immediate risks, including slightly increased rates of neonatal jaundice and the development of EPS in the newborn. These symptoms are transient and easily treated if they occur. After delivery, patients can return to taking antipsychotics, although the medications are certainly secreted in breast milk and can cause side effects in the infant if they breastfeed; most experts will discourage breastfeeding in such cases.

Neuromodulation

We have so far focused on pharmacological approaches to treating psychosis. However, there are other somatic therapies, loosely grouped under rubrics like "interventional psychiatry" or "neuromodulation." These approaches include treatments like ECT, rTMS, and tDCS. ECT has a long history in the treatment of psychotic disorders, but rTMS and tDCS are relatively newer, up and coming treatments that may play a greater role in the future as we learn more about how best to use them. Let us examine each of these treatments briefly.

ECT was developed by Italian psychiatrists Cerletti and Bini in the 1930s, originally for the treatment of schizophrenia. At the time, it was thought that seizures themselves might protect the brain from psychotic symptoms, because of observations made that patients with schizophrenia rarely had epilepsy (observations that turned out not to be accurate). For whatever reason, it seemed that patients who did have seizures (chemically induced or otherwise) experienced an improvement in their psychotic symptoms. There were few alternative treatments for patients with psychotic disorders, so when ECT emerged as a treatment, hospitals rapidly adopted it for their patients, and many were indeed helped with this intervention.

Over time, ECT became used more for other conditions (mood disorders and catatonia in particular), but it still appears to be effective for patients with psychotic disorders. Over a dozen research trials of nearly 900 patients with psychosis have consistently shown benefit from ECT, even in refractory states (with perhaps a 30% improvement rate overall, superior to anti-psychotic switches). Patients most likely to respond to ECT are those who have higher levels of mood or positive symptoms, who have catatonic features, who have had a recent onset of illness, or who require a rapid response (e.g., malnourished or aggressive patients).

Today, ECT's biggest role may be for clozapine partial responders or clozapine-resistant patients, to augment the medication. A 2015 study by Petrides et al., for instance, randomized 39 patients with schizophrenia to a single-blind eight-week protocol comparing clozapine alone to clozapine plus bilateral ECT (three times weekly for the first month, two times weekly thereafter). None of the control group responded, but 50% of those who received add-on ECT responded (defined as a 40% improvement in rating scales). Although there were some minor cognitive side effects, most patients tolerated the combination well.

There have been similar studies done by other groups, not just for clozapine/ECT but also for risperidone/ECT combinations. One of the challenges with this approach is the high relapse rate after discontinuation of ECT; maintenance or quick conversion to aggressive pharmacotherapy may be required to protect response. There are other challenges, of course, including lack of accessibility, stigma, and insurance coverage issues. And it is still not known how ECT actually works. But ECT is definitely appropriate as a treatment for psychotic disorders in specific situations.

A newer neuromodulation technique is rTMS, which had the opposite history of ECT: it was developed originally to treat depression and was later found to be somewhat helpful in psychosis. TMS uses wire coils to generate a targeted magnetic field, designed to trigger a smaller seizure with fewer side effects than seizures caused by ECT. It is also easier for practitioners to use. In a study by Zhao et al. (2014), 96 patients with schizophrenia or schizoaffective disorder were randomized to one of four rTMS protocols: sham, 10 hertz, 20 hertz, or theta burst stimulation. Treatments were given five days a week for a month, focusing on the left dorsolateral prefrontal cortex. The treatments were tolerable, with few dropouts and no major side effects; active treatment helped more than sham in reducing negative symptom burden. This result suggests that a symptom profile that has traditionally been hard to treat may yield to this new approach.

Furthermore, a review of rTMS by Slotema et al. (2014) examined 15 studies of 423 patients and found that low-frequency left temporoparietal cortex treatment improved refractory auditory hallucinations (effect size of about 40%, odds ratio of 2.94). There were no differences noted in negative or other symptoms. The only side effects noted were mild headache and facial muscle twitching; rTMS does not appear to have the cognitive side effects of ECT.

The differences in outcome raise questions about the overall role of rTMS in treating psychosis, and the treatment is not yet widely accessible. However, rTMS has been added to clinical guidelines (e.g., PORT, NICE) as an augmentation strategy for auditory hallucinations in psychotic disorders (Buchanan et al., 2010).

Finally, a new/old neuromodulation strategy is tDCS. Originally developed in the 1870s as "electrostimulation," tDCS was rediscovered by modern computer "gamers" hoping to gain a competitive advantage in performance. More recently, tDCS has been tried for patients with refractory auditory hallucinations, and two trials (120 patients) have been positive, especially for auditory verbal hallucinations. The treatment is administered by placing an anode on the left dorsolateral prefrontal cortex and a cathode over the temporoparietal cortex. The treatment is rapid, safe, and easy. Although the mechanism of action of tDCS is unknown, it may enhance neuroplasticity. At this point, tDCS is not included in clinical guidelines, but further research may bring it more to the fore.

Future Trends

In this chapter, we have explored the status of a variety of somatic therapy approaches to the treatment of psychosis. Some of these treatments date back a half-century or more, and some are relatively new. But our understanding of when and how to use these treatments is limited, and many symptoms respond poorly to existing treatments. In the coming decades, three broad trends are likely to influence the use of current treatments and help with the development of novel approaches to managing psychotic illness: translational neuroscience, personalized treatment, and phase-specific treatment.

First and most important, translational neuroscience promises a "ground-up" approach to therapeutic development. By learning more about brain functioning, and how the symptoms of psychosis are generated, we may be able to identify new targets for medication (e.g., glutamatergic treatments, the endocannabinoid system), or new approaches to specific symptom clusters (e.g., cognitive or negative symptoms). The NIMH has promulgated the Research Domain Criteria (RDoC) as a way of better organizing and directing neuroscience research into conditions like psychotic disorders, and this long-term approach may yield therapeutic fruit with time.

A second and perhaps related trend is the prospect of personalized treatment. For now, there is no way of predicting who will respond to what medication, or if someone is at higher risk for toxicity from specific medications. The rise of "psychogenomics," however, has led to the hope that we may someday have rational selection of treatment. For instance, recent work (Goldstein et al., 2014) has shown that individuals with specific genetic polymorphisms may be at much higher risk for developing clozapine-induced agranulocytosis; if individuals were tested for these polymorphisms in advance of a clozapine trial, it could enable very close observation, or promote a choice of alternate therapies, in those at highest risk. Other personalized treatment approaches may involve predicting metabolism of medications, identifying drug–drug interaction risks, or identifying specific dopamine-receptor targets in individuals.

Finally, more and more work is examining how treatments work in different phases of the illness (e.g., prodromal vs. maintenance phases). As more effectiveness research is done, we may have clearer ideas about phase-specific approaches: when to use clozapine, which antipsychotic is best in first-episode illness, and how medications combine with psychosocial treatments at different illness stages.

Other trends are likely to affect the somatic therapy pipeline, including new drug development (e.g., partial dopamine agonists, serotonergic medications), deep brain stimulation, and other neuromodulatory approaches. It is most likely, however, that a combination of approaches may allow a more individualized, pathophysiologically based approach to both diagnosis and treatment strategies.

Conclusion

Somatic treatments have long been a mainstay of care for individuals with psychotic disorders such as schizophrenia. ECT ended an era of therapeutic nihilism in psychiatry, giving hope to patients and families that recovery might be possible. Antipsychotics, developed in the 1950s, were discovered serendipitously but helped create the worldwide psychopharmacology industry of today and contributed to deinstitutionalization and the rise of community psychiatry, changing the way patients are treated and psychiatrists practice. Although these revolutionary therapies have been powerful and influential, and are an essential part of the care for individuals with psychotic disorders, they also have their limits in terms of their efficacy and toxicity. Treatment-refractory patients have pushed providers to try a host of polypharmacy/augmentation strategies, despite risks and limited data; clozapine remains the best choice for such individuals but is difficult to use. Managing side effects in general remains an essential part of care, and different treatment strategies are needed by phase of illness and for different populations. Future trends in somatic therapies for psychosis may help us develop better treatments for broader symptoms, treatments that can be better targeted to specific individuals at the most appropriate times.

Self-Learning Questions

1. Atypical (second-generation) antipsychotics primarily serve as antagonists to what neurotransmitter system(s)?
   a. Serotonin
   b. Dopamine
   c. Norepinephrine
   d. a and b
   e. All of the above

2. You have a patient for whom you would like to prescribe olanzapine. The patient asks about how the new medication compares to her last medication, haloperidol. What is the best response?
   a. Olanzapine has more risk for metabolic syndrome (elevated glucose, weight gain, etc.) and less risk of extrapyramidal symptoms (EPS including Parkinsonism, hyperprolactinemia, tardive dyskinesia).
   b. Olanzapine has less risk for metabolic syndrome and more risk for EPS.
   c. Olanzapine has the same general risk for both metabolic syndrome and EPS.
   d. Olanzapine has more risk for metabolic syndrome and the same risk for EPS.
   e. Olanzapine has the same risk for metabolic syndrome and less risk for EPS.

3. A 31-year-old male with schizoaffective disorder who was given fluphenazine (Prolixin), fluoxetine (Prozac) and Motrin complains of stiffness in his neck and jaw. A moment later he grasps his neck and begins choking. The most appropriate first treatment step is:
   a. Intramuscular benztropine (Cogentin)
   b. Intramuscular fluphenazine (Prolixin)
   c. Intravenous phenytoin (Dilantin)
   d. Intravenous carbamazepine (Tegretol)
   e. Intravenous gabapentin (Neurontin)

4. A 35-year-old man is transferred from another hospital because of intractable hallucinations. He has increasingly withdrawn from himself socially because of voices criticizing him and commanding him to "end it all." Several medications, including fluphenazine, haloperidol, olanzapine, and

perphenazine, have not helped. He is currently on risperidone 6 mg per day. The next step in management of this patient is:

a. Switch to quetiapine
b. Supplemental treatment with lithium
c. Increase the dose of risperidone
d. Consider instituting clozapine
e. Discontinue all medications and monitor closely

5. For refractory auditory hallucinations, unresponsive to clozapine, what might be the best neuromodulation option currently, based on treatment studies and guidelines?

a. Deep brain stimulation (DBS)
b. Repetitive transcranial magnetic stimulation (rTMS)
c. Unilateral electroconvulsive therapy (ECT)
d. Vagal nerve stimulation (VNS)

6. Dopamine antagonism is the primary mechanism of most antipsychotics; which one instead works primarily as a partial agonist at the D2 receptor?

a. Aripiprazole
b. Chlorpromazine
c. Fluphenazine
d. Lurasidone
e. Quetiapine

7. You have a patient who is very concerned about side effects, particularly both metabolic and movement, and would like you to pick an antipsychotic that has the lowest risk of such side effects. Of the following choices, which agent might be the safest option in this patient?

a. Clozapine
b. Haloperidol
c. Perphenazine
d. Quetiapine
e. Ziprasidone

Key Learning Points

• Antipsychotics are one part of a broad, disease-management approach for managing psychosis, but are an essential part of the biopsychosocial treatment for psychotic disorders, working particularly well in treating positive symptoms acutely, and for relapse prevention. Maintenance treatment is usually required.

• Significant toxicity, particularly movement and metabolic side effects, limit antipsychotic tolerability, acceptance, and use; this often leads to non-adherence, a major issue with this class of medication. Aggressive side-effect management is key, including ongoing monitoring.

• Second-generation antipsychotics have fewer movement side effects but more metabolic side effects, and are generally more expensive, without being any more efficacious.

• Clozapine is the only antipsychotic to demonstrate superior efficacy in treatment-refractory psychosis.

• Antipsychotic polypharmacy is not uncommon, but few combinations have shown any efficacy advantage, while all are costlier and risk more side effects. Augmentation with other psychotropics may have some promise for select symptoms.

• Neuromodulatory strategies like ECT can help in refractory psychosis, although more research needs to be done to fully assess them.

• Treatment must be carefully individualized by patient population and phase of illness to insure best outcomes.

• Research on personalized medicine and translational neuroscience may yield more effective approaches in the future.

References

American Diabetes Association, American Psychiatric Association, et al. (2004). Consensus development conference on antipsychotic drugs and obesity and diabetes. *Diabetes Care*, 27, 596–601.

American Psychiatric Association. (2004). Practice guidelines for the treatment of patients with schizophrenia. Second edition. *American Journal of Psychiatry*, 3(Suppl), 1–114.

Buchanan, R. W., Kreyenbuhl, J., et al. (2010). The 2009 schizophrenia PORT psychopharmacological treatment recommendations and summary statements. *Schizophrenia Bulletin*, 36, 71–93.

Carpenter, W. T., Buchanan, R. W., et al. (1999). Comparative effectiveness of fluphenazine decanoate injections every 2 weeks versus every 6 weeks. *American Journal of Psychiatry*, 156, 412–418.

Devinsky, O., Honigfeld, G., & Patin, J. (1991). Clozapine-related seizures. *Neurology*, 41, 369–371.

Goldstein, J. I., Jarskog, L. F., et al. (2014). Clozapine-induced agranulocytosis is associated with rare HLA-DQB1 and HLA-B alleles. *Nature Communications*, 5, 4757.

Harrigan, E. P., Miceli, J. J., et al. (2004). A randomized evaluation of the effects of six antipsychotic agents on QTc, in the absence and presence of metabolic inhibition. *Journal of Clinical Psychopharmacology*, 24, 62–69.

Jones, P. B., et al. (2006). Randomized controlled trial of the effect on quality of life of second- vs. first-generation antipsychotic drugs in schizophrenia: Cost Utility of the Latest Antipsychotic Drugs in Schizophrenia Study (CUtLASS 1). *Archives of General Psychiatry*, 32, 715–723.

Kane, J., Honigfeld, G., et al. (1988). Clozapine for the treatment-resistant schizophrenic: A double-blind comparison with chlorpromazine. *Archives of General Psychiatry*, 45, 789–796.

Leucht, S., Corves, C., et al. (2009). Second-generation versus first-generation antipsychotic drugs for schizophrenia: A meta-analysis. *Lancet*, 373, 31–41.

Lieberman, J. A., Stroup, T. S., et al. (2005). Effectiveness of antipsychotic drugs in patients with chronic schizophrenia. *New England Journal of Medicine*, 353, 1209–1223.

Maust, D. T., Kim, H. M., et al. (2015). Antipsychotics, other psychotropics, and the risk of death in patients with dementia: Number needed to harm. *Journal of the American Medical Association: Psychiatry*, 72, 438–445.

McEvoy, J. P., Lieberman, J. A., et al. (2006). Effectiveness of clozapine versus olanzapine, quetiapine, and risperidone in patients with chronic schizophrenia who did not respond to prior antipsychotic treatment. *American Journal of Psychiatry*, 163, 600–610.

McEvoy, J. P. (2006). Risks versus benefits of different types of long-acting injectable antipsychotics. *Journal of Clinical Psychiatry*, 67(Suppl 5), 15–18.

Meltzer, H. Y., et al. (2003). Serotonin receptors: Their key role in drugs to treat schizophrenia. *Progress in Neuro-Psychopharmacology and Biological Psychiatry*, 27, 1159–1172.

Mokhtari, M., & Rajarethinam, R. (2013). Early intervention and the treatment of prodrome in schizophrenia: A review of recent developments. *Journal of Psychiatric Practice*, 19, 375–385.

Moore, T. A., Buchanan, R. W., Buckley, P. F., Chiles, J. A., Conley, R. R., Crismon, M. L., et al. (2007). The Texas Medication Algorithm Project antipsychotic algorithm for schizophrenia: 2006 update. *Journal of Clinical Psychiatry*, 68, 880–887.

NICE. (2014). National collaborating centre for mental health, psychosis and schizophrenia in adults: treatment and management. *Clinical Guidelines, 178*. (https://www.nice.org.uk/guidance/cg178). Accessibility verified June 2016.

Petrides, G., Malur, C., et al. (2015). Electroconvulsive therapy augmentation in clozapine-resistant schizophrenia: A prospective, randomized study. *American Journal of Psychiatry, 172*, 52–58.

Robinson, G. E. (2012). Treatment of schizophrenia in pregnancy and postpartum. *Journal of Population Therapeutics and Clinical Pharmacology, 19*, e380–e386.

Rummel-Kluge, C., Komossa, K., et al. (2010). Head-to-head comparisons of metabolic side effects of second generation antipsychotics in the treatment of schizophrenia: A systemic review and meta-analysis. *Schizophrenia Research, 123*, 225–233.

Sikich, L., et al. (2008). Double-blind comparison of first- and second-generation antipsychotics in early-onset schizophrenia and schizoaffective disorder: Findings from the Treatment of Early-Onset Schizophrenia Spectrum Disorders (TEOSS) study. *American Journal of Psychiatry, 165*, 1420–1431.

Slotema, C. W., Blom, J. D., et al. (2014). Review of the efficacy of transcranial magnetic stimulation for auditory verbal hallucinations. *Biological Psychiatry, 76*, 101–110.

Stroup, T. S., et al. (2006). Effectiveness of olanzapine, quetiapine, risperidone, and ziprasidone in patients with chronic schizophrenia following discontinuation of a previous atypical antipsychotic. *American Journal of Psychiatry, 163*(4), 611–622.

Tauscher, J., Jones, C., et al. (2002). Significant dissociation of brain and plasma kinetics with antipsychotics. *Molecular Psychiatry, 7*, 317–321.

The International Psychopharmacology Algorithm Project. (2005). Available at http://www.ipap.org/. Accessibility verified June 2016.

Weiden, P. J., Citrome, L., et al. (2014). A trial evaluating gradual- or immediate-switch strategies from risperidone, olanzapine, or aripiprazole to iloperidone in patients with schizophrenia. *Schizophrenia Research*, 153–160–8.

Zhao, S., Kong, J., et al. (2014). Randomized controlled trial of four protocols of repetitive transcranial magnetic stimulation for treating the negative symptoms of schizophrenia. *Shanghai Archives of Psychiatry, 26*, 15–21.

Psychosocial Treatment for Psychotic Disorders: Systems of Care and Empirically Supported Psychosocial Interventions

Jessica M. Gannon and Shaun M. Eack

Introduction

The optimal treatment of schizophrenia and related psychotic disorders consists of appropriate antipsychotic pharmacotherapy integrated with psychosocial treatments designed to reduce vulnerability to stress and address social and vocational outcomes not targeted by current molecular approaches. Spurred on by early advances in psychopharmacology and increasing demands for deinstitutionalization, over the past 50 years, a large evidence base has developed supporting the psychosocial treatment for schizophrenia (Dixon et al., 2009; Mueser, Deavers, Penn, & Cassisi, 2013), ranging from basic supportive psychotherapies to advanced cognitive remediation approaches to address untreated impairments in cognitive function. These interventions are increasingly delivered within systems of care that focus on patient-centered goals of meaningful recovery.

In this chapter, we aim to:

1. Review the systems of care through which mental health interventions are delivered, ideally at levels of intensity tailored toward each patient's ongoing, and often changing, needs.

2. Provide an overview of psychosocial treatments for schizophrenia, including those tailored to address significant challenges to community integration, which often go beyond symptom management.

3. Address some of the challenges and special treatment considerations providers must consider when successfully working with individuals with schizophrenia and related psychotic disorders.

Before we begin this chapter, we would like to provide some brief clarifications as to terminology. In the following pages, individuals with schizophrenia and related psychotic disorders are most commonly referred to as "patients," but at times they may be alternatively termed "clients" or "mental health consumers." Such differences in nomenclature are common in the mental health field, with individuals from different educational and sociocultural backgrounds preferring different terminology in describing persons with mental illness. We would stress that, when labels are to be used to describe people, it is most important to consult the individual to whom the label will be applied to determine which label would be most agreeable. There are strong historical, and often personal, connotations associated with words like patient, and even client, that should be taken into consideration when administering person-centered care.

Within this chapter, you will also find multiple references to "recovery." The concept of recovery, as championed by many mental health consumer advocates, should not be confused with a medical or scientific standard of recovery. Here, recovery is seen as a process, not an outcome (Anthony, 1993), and it importantly focuses on coping and resilience more than on symptom elimination. There are goals in recovery, and they are consumer driven, highly individualized, strength-based, and embrace social connectedness and empowerment (Substance Abuse and Mental Health Services Administration [SAMHSA], 2005). The movement to make recovery the prime directive in mental health treatment probably began in the 1980s as a response to the often paternalistic and frequently negativist treatment models of the time (Bellack, 2006), and by 2002, the President's New Freedom Commission on Mental Health had supported the idea that the message of recovery be standard in mental health care (Hogan, 2003). The "recovery movement" has thus highly influenced all areas of mental health treatment, calling on clinicians to instill hope, while insisting that consumers and their families be approached with respect and as collaborative partners in treatment.

Systems of Care

Psychiatric care can be said to occur in one of two settings—inpatient or outpatient. For many seriously mentally ill individuals, particularly those with schizophrenia and related psychotic disorders, treatment was, until relatively recently, largely provided within inpatient hospitals. Many people with schizophrenia spent much of their lives living in such hospitals, which were designed for long-term care. Today, most people with schizophrenia receive their psychiatric services from providers who largely practice in outpatient settings. Both settings provide a wide array of services, offered to patients as per their individual treatment needs, and as described below.

Inpatient Hospitalization

Over the past several decades, long-term treatment of people with schizophrenia has gradually shifted from institutional settings to the community at large. Large psychiatric institutions, including the once-ubiquitous state mental hospitals, are seen as increasingly anachronistic to many in the broader mental health community. The closure of many such hospitals began with the implementation of the 1963 Community Mental Health Act, passed during the Kennedy administration in the wake of widespread concerns about the ethics of "warehousing" the mentally ill in institutions. Cost considerations are also a factor in this movement. Deinstitutionalization continues to be a controversial topic, with most agreeing that there are many benefits of treating patients in a community setting, including the promotion of patient self-efficacy and autonomy and social inclusion. Today's standard in psychiatric care is to treat patients in the least restrictive setting possible, helping to safeguard patients' civil liberties and personal freedoms. At the same time, many worry about the all-too-common gap in community services patients and their families have faced in the wake of deinstitutionalization. Many have linked the closure of state hospitals to the epidemic of homelessness and the incarceration of seriously mentally ill individuals, arguing that existing community treatment options are either underfunded and/or otherwise unequipped to respond to challenges in treatment of this population.

With continuing deinstitutionalization, hospitalization today is often reserved for the urgent periods of time when patients' needs cannot be adequately met by available outpatient programming. Hospitalizations, when they occur, are generally time-limited and ideally provide a safe, highly structured and supportive environment for treatment of patients who are struggling with significant symptom exacerbation and are considered to be in the acute stage of their illness. It is usually necessary for patients to be hospitalized when they pose an imminent and serious risk to their own safety or to the safety of others. Hospitalization can also be an invaluable resource for patients who are unable to adequately care for themselves during periods of symptoms exacerbation, requiring constant supervision and support to meet medical or nutritional needs. For seriously mentally ill patients in particular, inpatient hospitalization can allow for close observation of patients' current symptoms, enabling both diagnostic clarification and monitoring for effectiveness and side effects of often-complex medication regimens. If hospitalization is needed, and a patient is able to meaningfully consent to treatment, voluntary hospitalization should always be offered before involuntary means of hospitalization are pursued. Involuntary civil commitments to inpatient psychiatric facilities are available nationwide through each state, but vary in their criteria, duration, and enforcement. This will be discussed in further detail later in this chapter.

State mental hospitals and similar institutions still exist in many parts of the country, and such programs within the forensic or criminal justice system are more commonplace. In these institutions, the challenge continues to be to provide evidence-based, person-centered care, and generally speaking, patient discharge and reintegration in the community are now the standard goals of treatment. Unless the patients are legally sentenced to these institutions or otherwise remanded to their care, lengths of hospitalization still tend to be much shorter at long-term-stay psychiatric hospitals than in previous decades. Put another way, state hospitals increasingly focus on treating patients through the stabilization phase of illness rather than providing more stable phase treatment.

Outpatient Treatment
Long-Term Care Facilities
While many hospitals that traditionally provided long-term care for persons with serious mental illness have been closed, there remains a subpopulation of individuals with serious mental illness, particularly treatment-resistant schizophrenia, who more chronically require intensive and highly structured care. Some

states and various mental health agencies have had success with treating those with such significant illness burden in long-term structured residences, residential treatment facilities, and similar programs in community settings. The services provided in these places approach those of hospital-based care. Such facilities allow patients to be treated in a highly structured, safe environment with on-site physician and nursing staff. Patients in the stabilization phase of illness may be referred to these programs to gain additional clinical stability after an acute hospitalization, and also when they continue to require the time and significant support to gain the level of stability necessary for more complete community integration. Length-of-stay guidelines exist for many of these programs.

Day and Partial Hospitalizations
and Intensive Outpatient Treatment
Day hospitalization programs, when available, can sometimes be used as an alternative to acute inpatient hospitalization. With day hospitalizations, patients are provided with the same resources as an inpatient program affords, but they return to their usual place of residence in the evening. As such, collaboration with patients' housing staff, families, or other social supports promoting community living is integral for successful treatment planning in day hospitalization. There is evidence to suggest that day hospitalization can be a cost-effective way to reduce the need for inpatient hospitalization while providing effective treatment (Marshall et al., 2003). Partial hospitalizations and intensive outpatient programs may function similarly in providing a structured setting for patients at high risk for psychiatric decompensation, including during the period directly following an inpatient stay. The level of services provided by such programs varies in intensity and usually includes psychotherapy groups and peer support elements.

Crisis Programs
The aim of crisis intervention is to expediently address signs and symptoms of impending psychiatric decompensation by providing intense and time-limited treatment in a community setting. Interventions can include brief psychotherapies and medication, as well as family support. Participation is generally voluntary, and services are offered 24 hours a day and 365 days a year. A recent Cochrane review on these models of care, which included eight randomized controlled trials, demonstrated that hospitalization

rates were lower at six-month post-crisis intervention when compared to controls (Murphy et al., 2012). Family burden was also lower six months out, and patient satisfaction was higher in the intervention group at the 20-month follow-up. There were no significant differences in suicide attempt rates or death rates between groups.

While the goal of crisis intervention programs can be to help patients avoid inpatient hospitalization, clinicians in these programs are often called upon to help determine the most appropriate level of care for at risk patients. Mobile crisis teams, crisis residential programs, respites, crisis day programs, and even psychiatric emergency rooms and specialized crisis inpatient hospitalization units may operate under this model of care (Allen et al., 2002). Generally, goals of clinical stabilization include linkage to, or enhanced collaboration with, longer-term treatment providers.

Office-Based Outpatient Treatment
Traditional outpatient treatment is often based in an office, where patients go to attend appointments with a psychiatrist, and oftentimes, a therapist. Some outpatient treatment venues also employ other mental health providers, including physician assistants or nurse practitioners. Appointment duration and frequency are highly variable and dependent on patient preference, need, and resource availability. In most outpatient models, the psychiatrist will often serve as the head of the psychiatric treatment team and will also be called upon to collaborate with other medical doctors in care of the patient. Some outpatient sites offer integrated medical services as a part of a Health Home or similar model (SAMHSA-HRSA, 2012). Such service integration has been shown to increase the quality of medical care and improve health outcomes for people with serious mental illness (Druss et al., 2001). This is particularly important given this population's high rates of medical comorbidity. Outpatient programs may also offer specialty medication programs. These programs can include nursing and or pharmacy support for medications such as clozapine, which requires regular and frequent laboratory monitoring, and long-acting injectable (LAI) antipsychotics.

Psychiatric Rehabilitation
Psychiatric rehabilitation began, in the wake of deinstitutionalization, to promote community integration of the seriously mentally ill, providing services designed to meet the needs of

individuals who had been institutionalized over significant portions of their lives (Cohen, Farkas, & Gange, 2002). Many former patients discharged from institutions found that they did not know how to live outside of the rigid structure of a hospital, and the communities into which they were released were not always welcoming. Psychiatric rehabilitation in its modern form was largely disseminated from several large academic centers, including Boston University's Rehabilitation Research and Training Center on Psychiatric Rehabilitation.

Psychiatric rehabilitation today works to teach and foster, in patients with serious mental illness, the skills they need to be members of the communities of their choosing. Challenges of community integration remain for seriously mentally ill patients, especially individuals with schizophrenia, as symptoms of the disorder itself, as well as the social stigma and poverty too often associated with the disorder, can negatively affect patients' ability to work, go to school, live independently, and build meaningful relationships. Psychiatric rehabilitation strategies remain crucial in the effective treatment of the seriously mentally ill; therefore, their influence can be found in many domains of psychosocial service delivery, like traditional outpatient clinics and housing programs, and in psychosocial treatments themselves, including vocational rehabilitation programs and Assertive Community Treatment (ACT) teams (please see later in this chapter). The Clubhouse movement, in which involved persons are called "members," not patients or clients, is a form of psychiatric rehabilitation that generally operates outside of traditional mental health models (e.g., does not involve psychiatrists or therapists).

Psychiatric rehabilitation differentiates itself from other described treatment delivery systems in that it does not focus on the relief of psychiatric symptoms. Psychiatric rehabilitation focuses instead on improving role functioning, helping the patient achieve personal goals in vocational, educational, residential, social, and familial domains. Many practices common to psychiatric rehabilitation, such as social skills training and vocational rehabilitation (both explored later in this chapter), have a strong evidence base for efficacy. As a whole, psychiatric rehabilitation facilitates a person's identifying personal strengths and skills to better reach or keep their recovery goals. It approaches people with respect and facilitates empowerment and hope as integral to treatment (Anthony & Farkas, 2009).

Psychosocial Interventions

The modern era has brought with it myriad promising psychosocial interventions in treating individuals with schizophrenia and related psychotic disorders. Many of these modalities are widely available, while others are less commonly encountered. All of the practices detailed below are supported by an evidence base, and many continue to evolve to work to best meet the needs of patients.

While the impact of psychosocial interventions on the outcome of patients with schizophrenia can be great, a word of caution is advised. An early lesson learned by interventionists stressed the fundamental need for antipsychotic treatment. As expected, patients randomized to chlorpromazine and sociotherapy had far better outcomes than those receiving chlorpromazine alone (Hogarty et al., 1974a), but those assigned to sociotherapy and placebo fared worse on many outcomes than those receiving placebo alone (Hogarty et al., 1974b). This key finding highlights both the critical need to integrate antipsychotic treatment into the application of psychosocial treatments and the potential for intense psychotherapies to hamper treatment response in the absence of pharmacotherapy. Clearly, optimal treatment consists of a combination of medication and psychosocial treatment modalities, generally with overarching goals of promoting community integration and recovery.

Case Management

Patients with schizophrenia frequently benefit from, and sometimes require, support from multiple service providers to maintain successful mental health treatment and community integration. Case management is a model called upon by many mental health agencies to help ensure that patients receive coordinated, comprehensive care often delivered in varying treatment settings. Case managers work with their clients to identify and link them to resources that will help them achieve specific goals. They can be essential in helping patients navigate complex systems involving housing, vocational opportunities, disability benefits, and medical insurance. Case managers also play an important role in facilitating communication between their client, his or her psychiatric treatment team members, and the client's natural supports. Depending on the model of case management, some case managers meet with clients in a designated space, often in an office, while others meet with their clients in a community setting of the clients' choosing. Some case managers specialize in assisting specific types of clients, such as those with forensic or substance use issues. In many mental health agencies, there also exist different "levels," or intensities, of case management services based on client need and service availability. Case management, particularly of a more intense variety, in which smaller client caseloads per case manager are maintained, may reduce lengths of hospitalization and increase patient retention in care (Dieterich et al., 2010). It should be noted that in some systems, terms like "service coordinator" may be used in lieu of "case manager," as the term "case manager" is not always perceived as person-centered or recovery-oriented.

Assertive Community Treatment

Assertive Community Treatment, or ACT, is a specialized program in which intensive case management and psychiatric treatment interventions are highly integrated to serve patients in a community setting. This evidence-based mental health intervention has repeatedly been shown to reduce hospitalization as well as increase housing stability, which can be a significant concern and is explored later in this chapter (National Alliance on Mental Illness [NAMI], 2007). ACT teams include at least one psychiatrist, nurses, and multiple clinicians, and the caseload of patients served is kept relatively small. Clinicians on an ACT team may have specific areas of expertise, which can include a specialization in forensics, drug and alcohol counseling, or vocational training. Certified peer specialists, or self-identified mental health consumers who have received specialized training and certification in providing recovery-oriented mental health services, are often integrated into ACT teams as well.

Patients may be referred to ACT teams after having been identified as requiring significant support to avoid repeated inpatient hospitalization, incarceration, or homelessness. In many mental health systems, the patients referred to ACT teams are frequent, high utilizers of psychiatric care. While ACT teams often serve patients with multiple diagnoses, the program was originally designed for persons with serious mental illness who struggled with community integration upon de-institutionalization (Stein & Test, 1980). Treatment plan goals in ACT are patient-centered and generally aim to maximize patients' social and vocational functioning. These goals can range from tasks as fundamental as a patient's mastering basic hygiene skills, to handling more complex responsibilities, like budgeting personal finances. Assistance with medication administration is also frequently offered. Treatment itself generally occurs in patients' homes, places of work, or other community settings. ACT teams offer services 24 hours a day, seven days a week, and are active in crisis situations.

Housing Programs

Housing options and resources for people with serious mental illness, including those with psychotic spectrum disorders, are varied. A person-centered approach to helping patients achieve suitable housing is recommended. Psychiatric care and support are an integral aspect of some of housing options, while others may promote more autonomy and/or reliance on natural social supports.

Support for Independent and Family Living

Many seriously mentally ill individuals thrive in living independently, and like most people, they utilize social and natural supports as needed to maintain successful community integration. Others live in traditional family settings, with parents, siblings, or their own significant others and children, and with varying levels of assistance provided by these natural supports. Some patients' families might find themselves needing to be highly involved in multiple aspects of the identified patient's psychiatric care. Family psychoeducation programs can be very helpful in these situations (see Family Psychoeducation section below), as can membership in organizations like NAMI. Coping with and providing needed support for a family member with schizophrenia can be incredibly stressful, especially if the family is at odds with the patient concerning treatment. Ideally, families will be hands-on in their support when a patient is more acutely ill but will encourage the patient to demonstrate more autonomy when the patient is stable. Caretaker burnout is a real risk in caring for a loved one with a serious mental illness, and it is important for a patient's treatment team to recognize the stress that caring for a patient can place on the patient's natural supports.

Various voluntary services exist to help support people who live in these independent or familial settings, ranging from case management services to visiting psychiatric nurses. Availability of such services varies widely by region. Some of these services are directly linked to supported housing or other community integration programs.

Supported Housing

Supported housing programs offer a variety of services to assist individuals with mental health conditions in securing or maintaining community-integrated housing. Housing may be in one site, like in an apartment complex, or scattered throughout multiple sites. The overarching goal of supported housing is to promote the housing stability of individual, mentally ill persons. Services provided are voluntary, flexible in scope and intensity, and driven by consumer preference and need. Programs may incorporate rehabilitation, case management, and treatment elements. Some programs, for example, may offer meal-preparation training and budgeting support while simultaneously linking clients to mental health services and monitoring self-medication administration. Supported housing programs sometimes offer direct financial assistance to clients for rent payment, or they assist in linking clients with the federal Department of Housing and Urban Development (HUD), Section 8, or other government-subsidized housing.

The evidence base for the efficacy of supported housing in housing retention, often exceeding 80% in studies, as well as in decreased time spent in acute mental health settings, continues to expand (Rogers, Kash-MacDonald, & Olschewski, 2009). Supported housing is a key component of the widely known Housing First initiatives, first implemented in the early 1990s by Dr. Sam Tsemberis and Pathways to Housing in New York City. Their projects and associated research focused on chronically homeless and dually diagnosed individuals. Unlike in a traditional housing model, in which clients have to be actively engaged in mental health treatment and/or treatment for substance use disorders, clients engaged in Housing First programs were offered housing without having to commit to treatment. In Dr. Tsemberis's work, Housing First clients not only were able to retain housing at a high rate, but they also largely chose to be involved in mental health treatment (Tsemberis & Eisenberg, 2000).

Residential Care Facilities

Residential care facilities provide supported housing integrated with mental health services. Since the deinstitutionalization movement of the 1960s, the goal of many types of residential care facilities has been to promote community integration and functional independence of individuals with serious mental illness. At its most basic, this type of housing provides residents with room and board and varying levels of assistance in activities of daily living, as well as supervised medication administration. In more intensive programs, the care provided may also include individual and group psychotherapy, psychiatric rehabilitation services, and care by a psychiatrist. Acceptance of psychiatric treatment is often a prerequisite for residents living in this type of housing. Residential care facilities can be state-run or operated by nonprofit or, less commonly, for-profit, organizations. They are generally licensed and regulated by state governments, and the type and scope of facilities in existence vary broadly among states. Residential care facilities feature a wide variety of more specific housing types, and can include adult residential facilities, adult foster homes, community care homes, group homes, domiciliary homes, and personal care homes, among others (Fleishman, 2004). Some cater to specific populations, including the dually diagnosed or patients with forensic issues. Other homes may cater to the elderly. It should be noted, though, that nursing homes are not considered residential care facilities, in that nursing homes provide essential nursing care for individuals who are significantly medically compromised and at high risk for frequent medical hospitalization without such care. Some nursing homes, however, do cater to individuals with coexisting serious medical and mental illness.

Residential care facilities most often differentiate themselves based on the intensity of services provided, with higher intensity programs tailored to patients with more complex or extensive treatment needs. They may also be classified by anticipated resident length of stay, with some facilities offering permanent housing options. Time-limited programs that are simultaneously highly service-intensive often treat seriously mentally ill patients on referral from an acute inpatient hospital, with the goal of helping the patients gain additional clinical stability after an acute hospitalization. These programs allow patients to be treated in a highly structured, safe environment, generally with on-site physicians and nursing staff. Patients are ultimately discharged to a variety of outpatient housing options, ideally based on their clinical need and the presence or absence of natural supports.

Facilities that fall within the "transitional housing paradigm" provide services for a time-limited period but tend to cater to individuals who are less severely impaired at the time of admission. Many of these programs will have discharge goals, tailored for each patient, and strive to prepare residents for independent living. Residents generally live in transitional housing with decreasing levels of formal support as they advance in their recovery (Lehman et al., 2004). Other facilities have longer lengths of stay and can become permanent residences as needed.

Programs that offer longer term care generally target more psychiatrically stable patients. Group homes, personal care homes, adult care homes, and domiciliary care homes often fall into this category of residential care facility (Figure 7.1). As many institutions that traditionally provided long-term care for persons with serious mental illness have been closed, this type of community-based, long-term residential care has been increasingly called upon to provide housing for a subpopulation of individuals with serious mental illness, particularly treatment-resistant schizophrenia. Housing for such individuals has remained a challenge for many states and mental health agencies, as programs that provide extensive and comprehensive support may not always be readily available. As such, some states have faced harsh criticism for housing individuals with serious mental illness in long-term care facilities that were inadequate for their needs (Marx & Jackson, 2012) (*New York Times*, 2002).

Psychotherapeutic Approaches

Psychotherapy is fundamental in the treatment of mental illness, including schizophrenia. Here, we discuss some of the most commonly utilized, as well as some of the most promising, psychotherapies for the treatment of schizophrenia.

Supportive Therapy

Supportive therapy is a cornerstone of psychosocial treatment for many mental disorders, and schizophrenia and psychotic disorders are no exception. Supportive therapy approaches vary widely, but all generally consist of the provision of a skilled empathic therapist trained in the use of active listening, making supportive comments, and developing a therapeutic relationship with the patient. Some include aspects of stress management and relaxation training, others emphasize medication management, and still others largely focus on developing the therapeutic relationship and view that as an essential treatment target. Decades of psychotherapy research have indicated that these "non-specific" elements of therapy may in fact be considerable drivers of treatment benefit for many patients (Messer & Wampold, 2002).

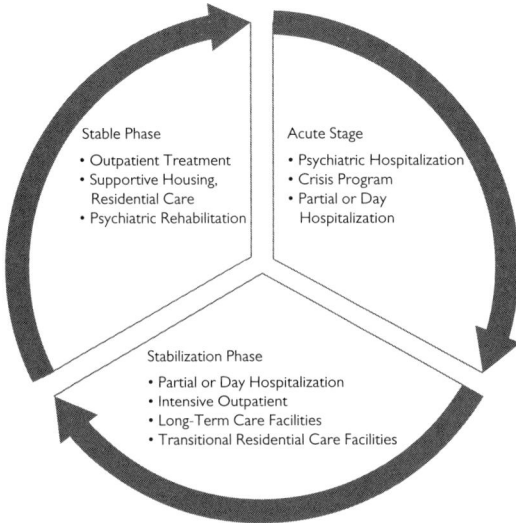

Figure 7.1 *Systems of care and stages of illness*: Many treatment modalities target treatment to specific illness stages. A patient may benefit from, or even require, hospitalization during a psychotic decompensation. Some patients, however, may be diverted from hospitalization through use of crisis program and/or intensive outpatient services, like partial hospitalization. Patients in the stabilization phase may require intensive services in a clinical and/or residential setting. Stable patients receive services in a wide variety of settings, which may incorporate a psychiatric rehabilitation focus. Many psychotherapeutic treatment interventions are beneficial throughout the illness course, including case management services and ACT teams. Like medication, psychotherapy is important in treating all phases of illness, with the intensity and focus of therapy varying with illness stage.

Although supportive therapy is rarely the focus of treatment trials in schizophrenia, these treatments are often used as the contrasting condition for a new experimental approach in research, given their widespread use in the field and generally agreed-upon benefits (Penn et al., 2004). As such, considerable data on their efficacy have emerged from the field. Studies have found that supportive therapies in schizophrenia can reduce positive symptoms (e.g., Penn et al., 2009), forestall relapse (e.g., Tarrier et al., 2000), and improve social adjustment (e.g., Hogarty et al., 2004). Although a recent meta-analysis found no benefits of supportive therapy over usual care for the treatment of schizophrenia (Buckley, Pettit, & Adams, 2007), it is likely that these findings reflect more the use of supportive therapy as usual care in much of the mental health community than a lack of efficacy of such approaches.

Given that supportive therapy is a cornerstone of community practice in the treatment of schizophrenia and related psychotic disorders, it is reassuring that the basic provision of a skilled therapist who can develop an empathic and supportive therapeutic relationship with patients can confer benefits to a variety of outcomes. It is important to remember, however, that supportive therapy is far from a standard model of care. There is great heterogeneity in what is implemented as supportive therapeutic practices, and the more effective approaches do seem to draw from aspects of cognitive-behavioral therapy, psychoeducation, and personal therapy (Penn et al., 2004). It is currently not known what the active mechanisms of such treatments are in schizophrenia, but it is likely that the development of the therapeutic relationship is necessary but not sufficient for meaningful change in symptom or functional outcomes in people with schizophrenia. Consequently, supportive therapy should represent a beginning approach to the psychosocial treatment of this population, which ultimately needs to progress to targeted and disorder-relevant approaches to provide the greatest opportunity for recovery.

Family Psychoeducation

One of the most effective and widely tested psychosocial approaches to the treatment of schizophrenia, beyond assertive community treatment (see "Psychiatric Rehabilitation," above), is family psychoeducation. This approach was developed in the late 1970s by Carol M. Anderson and Gerard E. Hogarty at the University of Pittsburgh, where they coined the term "psychoeducation" to refer to the education of individuals and their families about their own psychological health and disability (Anderson, Hogarty, & Reiss, 1980). The development of family psychoeducation came at a time when family members were not routinely educated about schizophrenia (and at times were actively excluded from knowing a patient's diagnosis), but were commonly the primary post-hospital caretakers for patients with the disorder. Previous work had demonstrated that the family environment was a strong predictor of psychotic relapse in patients, particularly environments that were characterized by high levels of criticism and emotional overinvolvement, otherwise known as "expressed emotion" (Butzlaff & Hooley, 1998). As a consequence, family psychoeducation was developed to help strengthen and support the family environment to adjust to the onset of schizophrenia. Anderson and Hogarty postulated that, by demystifying the illness and arming families with the latest information on what to expect from schizophrenia, they would enable families to adjust far better to being caretakers for their relatives and support the development of a low-stress family environment (Anderson, Reiss, & Hogarty, 1986). This hypothesis earned considerable early merit, demonstrating strikingly low levels of post-hospital relapse among patients receiving family psychoeducation (Hogarty et al., 1986; Hogarty et al., 1991), signifying the considerable benefits of including family members and educating them about schizophrenia.

Since Anderson and Hogarty's early work on family psychoeducation in schizophrenia, over 20 randomized controlled trials of the treatment have been conducted. Meta-analyses of this research suggest that rates of psychotic relapse can be reduced by 20% or more by providing family psychoeducation (Pitschel-Walz, Leucht, Bäuml, Kissling, & Engel, 2001). While rehospitalization and relapse are the most widely studied outcomes, others have demonstrated benefits to such far-reaching outcomes as medication adherence (McFarlane et al., 1995), positive symptoms (Rotondi et al., 2010), and family burden (Mueser et al., 2001; Xiong et al., 1994). As evidence has accumulated for the benefits of family psychoeducation in patients with schizophrenia, several models have become prominent. In addition to the traditional family psychoeducation model, multi-family group psychoeducation has shown considerable efficacy and become popular due to its efficient application in a group-based format (McFarlane et al., 1995). Another prominent model in community practice is NAMI's Family-to-Family program, which also has shown benefits (Dixon et al., 2001). These findings broadly suggest that many different modalities and methods for involving families in the treatment of schizophrenia can be effective. The most central components appear to be joining with families, teaching them problem-solving strategies, delivering education about the illness, and helping family members adjust to living with someone with a chronic disability. Meta-analytic reviews also indicate that long-term involvement is necessary for outcome improvement, as few gains are made for treatments shorter than six months in duration (Dixon et al., 2009).

Patient Psychoeducation

As effective as family psychoeducation has been shown to be, many have also recognized the importance of educating patients with schizophrenia about their condition and how to manage and make life adjustments accordingly. Patient psychoeducation was a focal point of many of the family psychoeducation models, including the original model by Anderson and Hogarty, but most models did not require this as a key component. Furthermore, for the patients not living with their family, it was even more crucial that they understood the nature of schizophrenia and how to support their own recovery.

Patient psychoeducation is very common in routine clinical practice and usually consists of providing the patient with information about schizophrenia and related psychotic disorders, including their early signs and symptoms, the role of stress in these conditions, the importance of medication and psychosocial treatment, and strategies to prevent relapse. There is no single model of patient psychoeducation, and rarely are such interventions the sole focus of efficacy trials, but rather education is integrated into broader, individual-based psychosocial treatment packages designed to facilitate illness management and prevent rehospitalization. One example of this approach is Personal Therapy (Hogarty, 2002), which is an individual-based approach divided into phases tailored to the level of recovery of the patient. In the basic phase, patients may still be stabilizing and learning relatively simple skills to manage their condition, such as avoiding stressful situations and using passive distraction techniques. As patients progress in their recovery, more advanced education and stress management approaches are learned, such as how to implement diaphragmatic breathing, detection and management of early prodromal signs, and managing criticism. One can easily see that this rich approach integrates aspects of skills training, relapse prevention, and relaxation training, all within an illness-management and psychoeducation approach, as is commonly done in patient psychoeducation interventions.

Evidence for the efficacy of patient psychoeducation alone is minimal (Lincoln, Wilhelm, & Nestoriuc, 2007), given that most studies evaluate the benefits of such an approach within larger treatment packages. Personal Therapy has shown considerable benefits in preventing relapse and improving long-term adjustment (Hogarty et al., 1997a; Hogarty et al., 1997b), as have many other "illness management and recovery" programs (Mueser et al., 2002). Overall, there is clear evidence for the benefits of psychoeducation treatments that are integrated with larger relapse-prevention programs for improving knowledge about schizophrenia and medication adherence, as well as reducing psychiatric symptomatology and rehospitalization (Mueser et al., 2002). Although intervention approaches that only provide patient psychoeducation may be helpful for increasing knowledge, they do not show clear benefits when used in isolation (Lincoln, Wilhelm, & Nestoriuc, 2007), and they clearly need to be integrated within broader treatment programs to support greater recovery.

Social Skills Training

The challenges in social functioning that patients with schizophrenia and other psychotic conditions experience are considerable and persist well beyond the remission of positive symptoms (Mueser, Bellack, Douglas, & Morrison, 1991; Mueser & Tarrier, 1998). Social skills training is one of the original approaches designed to address these problems in social functioning. This set of interventions is based largely on behaviorist principles of modeling, role-playing, and social learning (Bellack, Mueser, Gingerich, & Agresta, 2004; Wallace & Liberman, 1985). Most social skills training programs have a series of social skill modules that they focus on, ranging from basic conversation skills to job interviewing. Treatment usually consists of identifying the behavioral principles behind the social skill to be trained (e.g., for conversation skills: make eye contact, comment on the social context, and actively listen), modeling that skill, and then role-playing and practicing the particular skill in a therapeutic context until the patient develops a sufficient level of proficiency. This format has been applied to a large number of social and even illness-management skills under the umbrella of social skills training, since many specific skills can be broken down into their behavioral components relatively easily, which provides an attainable level of instruction for patients coping with challenging impairments.

There have been over 20 randomized controlled trials of social skills training for patients with schizophrenia, and the evidence is largely supportive of its efficacy for improving social and other skills in this population. A recent meta-analysis indicated large effects on skill acquisition and more moderate effects on community functioning (Kurtz & Mueser, 2008). There appears to be little benefit from this approach to psychotic symptoms or relapse, however (Hogarty et al., 1991), which might be expected, given that the approach does not generally target positive symptoms, although some versions do target skills (e.g., medication management) that are likely to have effects on symptomatology, if implemented. Social skills training has been diversely applied to both inpatient and outpatient populations with success, making it accessible to patients at different stages of their recovery. There has been some debate about the generalizability of skills practiced in the therapeutic setting to everyday places and activities (Wallace et al., 1980), and the difference in effect sizes between skill acquisition and community functioning does suggest a loss in implementing such skills in daily life. However, a balanced view would also indicate that some benefits to social and community functioning are clearly maintained (e.g., Marder et al., 1996). Overall, social skills training appears to be an effective behavioral approach to facilitating the acquisition of various social and daily living skills, which can facilitate functional recovery in people with schizophrenia.

Cognitive Behavior Therapy for Psychosis
Cognitive behavior therapy (CBT) for psychosis is a novel approach to addressing positive symptoms in schizophrenia that is based on the work of Aaron T. Beck in the development of cognitive therapy for depressive disorders (Beck, 1964). The fundamental principle of cognitive therapy is that psychopathology is the result of persistent distorted patterns of thinking that ultimately give rise to disorder and functional impairment, and that if patients are helped to recognize such cognitive disorders, they can thereby implement strategies to correct their thinking and alleviate at least some degree of associated symptomatology. This approach has been shown to be as, if not more, effective for the treatment of depression than pharmacotherapy (Butler, Chapman, Forman, & Beck, 2006), and in the past several decades it has been adapted for addressing the positive symptoms of schizophrenia. In adapting CBT for the psychotic population, the underlying principles and targets of cognitive

therapy have remained similar to its application in affective disorders. The primary target continues to be distorted and irrational thinking, except that this centers around delusional and paranoid thinking instead of depressive thoughts. These approaches are usually applied on an individual basis, although group-based efforts have been used, with the therapist and patient seeking a shared understanding of the cognitive basis of the patient's psychotic experiences. Explicit formulations are developed that situate these experiences around cognitive biases (e.g., identification of personalization bias in patients with paranoid delusions), and then dialogue and reality-testing experiments are developed to test the accuracy of these thoughts, with an effort to replace biased thinking with thoughts that more closely approximate reality. Furthermore, standard behavioral strategies, such as relaxation training and coping skills training, are implemented along with cognitive therapy approaches to help reduce distress caused by positive symptoms (Kingdon & Turkington, 1994).

Most of the research on CBT for psychosis has been conducted in Europe, particularly the United Kingdom, and the evidence base for the efficacy of these approaches has been strong enough to support widespread implementation by the National Health Service (NHS) for any person who has a diagnosis of schizophrenia. Currently, there are more than 30 randomized-controlled trials of CBT for psychosis, and evidence suggests that this approach can have a modest but significant benefit to both positive and negative symptoms (Jauhar et al., 2014). Stronger evidence does appear when used with patients with medication-resistant symptoms (Burns, Erickson, & Brenner, 2014), who demonstrate moderate reductions in positive and general psychopathology symptoms. Such findings are particularly compelling because patients who are medication-refractory by definition are not benefiting from antipsychotic treatment, and the challenge of reducing positive symptoms is therefore even greater in this population. Nearly all studies have focused on medicated patients, even if refractory, although a recent trial compared CBT for psychosis to usual care for patients who were refusing medication (Morrison et al., 2004). Results showed significant reductions in positive and general psychiatric symptoms in patients who received CBT for psychosis without medication compared to usual care without medication, suggesting that this approach may be beneficial for people who are refusing antipsychotic treatment. However, caution should be taken when considering this approach in lieu of medication, as serious adverse events (attempted suicide and homicidal behavior) did occur in several of the non-medicated CBT for psychosis patients, although the frequency of these incidents was less than with usual care. Taken together, such findings suggest that helping patients recognize and correct cognitive biases in their thinking is an effective approach for reducing the level of distress experienced due to positive symptoms, particularly for patients who refuse antipsychotic medication.

Supported Employment

Most individuals with schizophrenia have a desire to work; unfortunately, the disabling nature of the condition, the stigma associated with mental illness, and policies that disincentivize work make it exceedingly difficult for people with the disorder to obtain and maintain employment (Marwaha & Johnson, 2004). Per a recent report from NAMI, at least 80% of people with a serious mental illness are unemployed (Diehl, Douglas, Gay, & Hart, 2014). Employment rates in recent years also appear to be on the decline. Of serious mentally ill individuals who receive public mental health services, 23% were employed in 2003, compared to 17.8% in 2012. These numbers did vary greatly by state, as did the availability of vocational support services.

Supportive employment programs have been developed to address at least some of the challenges people with schizophrenia face in obtaining and maintaining employment. Such programs focus on helping individuals build the skills they need to re-enter the workforce with success. The most prevalent supported employment program with the largest evidence base is the Individual Placement and Support (IPS) program (Bond, 1998). The fundamental principles of IPS include a focus on competitive employment, instead of sheltered workshops or work set aside for patients; support and assessment in the actual work setting that is not time-limited; and the integration of mental health and vocational rehabilitation services. Rapid job attainment is also a central focus, as many consumers seem to be idle in perpetual pre-employment training, and one of the best ways to learn job skills is in an actual job. Furthermore, the work preferences of patients is a priority in job seeking, so the supportive employment counselors help them target their efforts toward areas of work that they find motivating, which are usually quite realistic. Individuals entering into a supportive employment program based on this model will receive a supportive employment counselor who is a vocational rehabilitation specialist that will help them build interviewing skills and target job opportunities, and will visit them on the job site to conduct work assessments and provide support.

Supported employment programs for improving employment outcomes for people with schizophrenia have received significant evaluation and support in the literature. There have been at least nine randomized controlled trials in patients with severe mental illness, and meta-analytic reviews indicate that, on average, such programs enable 51% of patients to find and obtain competitive employment, a rate that is four times that of those who do not receive supported employment (Bond, Drake, & Becker, 2008; Twamley, Jeste, & Lehman, 2003). In one large multi-site study conducted in Europe, investigators found that patients who received supportive employment worked significantly more hours, spent more days in work, and were less likely to be rehospitalized than individuals in traditional vocational rehabilitation programs (Burns et al., 2007). In a meta-analytic study of the efficacy of supported employment based on patient demographic and work history, results indicated little variability in efficacy, and the authors broadly concluded that such interventions were effective for a wide range of patients (Campbell, Bond, & Drake, 2011). Although some concerns have been raised about the long-term benefits of supportive employment in schizophrenia, results from multi-year follow-up studies do suggest that the benefits of these treatments to work can be maintained (Becker, Whitley, Bailey, & Drake, 2007).

Cognitive Remediation
In the past several decades, a new generation of approaches to the psychosocial treatment of schizophrenia has emerged that targets the pervasive cognitive impairments associated with the condition (Eack, 2012). Psychologists have observed for many years that people with schizophrenia experience considerable deficits in basic information-processing domains, such as attention, memory, and executive function (Heinrichs & Zakzanis, 1998), as well as areas of cognition that involve the processing of social information, such as understanding the perspectives of others and how social cues in the environment convey important information about appropriate behavior (Penn, Corrigan, Bentall, Racenstein, & Newman, 1997). Although pharmacological approaches to the treatment of these impairments have met with little success (Buchanan et al., 2007; Keefe et al., 2007),

psychosocial cognitive-remediation interventions are showing considerable promise. Cognitive remediation is based on principles of brain plasticity, which suggest that enriched environmental experiences can produce core neuronal changes that support increase cognitive efficiency and efficacy (Cramer & Riley, 2008). Many different approaches have been applied to patients with schizophrenia, ranging from repeated practice on paper-and-pencil cognitive tests to advanced computer- and group-based remediation interventions. The most common interventions utilize hands-off computer exercises designed to "work out" specific aspects of cognitive function that are hypothesized to be deficient, often using a drill-and-practice approach of repeated practice to improve mental stamina and cognitive abilities. Some approaches also make use of strategic training where individuals engage, not only in cognitive exercises, but also in explicit training in how to approach cognitive challenges with strategies that will improve their efficiency of processing and successful problem solving. Most interventions focus on neurocognitive abilities in attention, memory, or executive function, with fewer treatments available for impairments in social cognition. Cognitive enhancement therapy is the only cognitive remediation approach that targets social and non-social cognitive impairments in schizophrenia (Hogarty & Greenwald, 2006).

To date, there have been over 40 studies of cognitive remediation in schizophrenia, and meta-analytic reviews indicate significant and moderate effect size improvements in overall cognitive function among patients who received these treatments (Wykes et al., 2011). These improvements are greater than have been observed with medications alone, and importantly, they are also associated with significant improvements in functional outcome in some studies. Whether the approach is computer-based or paper-and-pencil based appears to make little difference in efficacy, but the studies that employ strategic training methods show greater levels of efficacy. In addition, significant benefits on functional outcome have been greater in studies that use comprehensive approaches to the treatment of social and non-social cognition (Hogarty et al., 2004; Eack et al., 2009) or integrate cognitive remediation with other psychiatric rehabilitation interventions (McGurk et al., 2007). Although there are comparatively fewer interventions that focus on social cognition, results from these studies do indicate significant benefits on a variety of social-cognitive domains (Kurtz & Richardson, 2012). Finally, evidence is also indicating that cognitive remediation interventions can protect against brain loss early in the course of the disorder (Eack et al., 2010) and enhance brain function in different neural systems (Subramaniam et al., 2012; Wykes et al., 2002).

Special Considerations in Psychosocial Treatment

In working with people with schizophrenia and related psychotic disorders, it is important to explore for the presence of specific comorbid psychiatric conditions, as well as certain social issues that may be particularly prevalent in this population. Treating substance use disorder is particularly important to the overall mental health of people with schizophrenia. Homelessness and incarceration are not uncommon treatment challenges in this population, and much attention should be given to providing evidence-based care when these arise.

A common challenge in working with people with schizophrenia is their refusal of voluntary treatment. Often, involuntary treatment of such individuals is, under very specific conditions, legally permissible. This type of treatment and some of the controversies inherent therein are explored in depth later in this chapter. Issues of meaningful consent to treatment may also arise periodically for some patients, usually during periods of psychiatric decompensation. The use of psychiatric advanced directives can be an empowering for patients who encounter these situations, and this topic is also discussed. Guardianship is also reviewed here, as this is a legal option that may be pursued when patients profoundly lack broader decision-making capacities.

Substance Use Disorders

Special treatment considerations should be given to individuals with comorbid schizophrenia and substance use disorders. The literature commonly cites an over 50% lifetime prevalence of substance use disorder in this population, not counting nicotine use, with the most common substances of abuse being alcohol and/or marijuana (Fowler et al., 1998; Soyka et al., 1992). Individuals with schizophrenia and co-occurring substance use disorder have been shown to have increased psychotic symptom severity, increased rates of hospitalization, decreased medication adherence, and poorer response to medication (Dixon, 1999). Other outcomes are also worse, including higher rates of perpetration of violence (Steadman et al., 1998) and increased homelessness (Dixon, 1999).

In treating people with schizophrenia spectrum and co-occurring substance use disorders, a comprehensive treatment model is generally recommended, in which treatment goals particular to schizophrenia and substance use disorder are simultaneously approached. Such programs might involve assertive outreach, staged interventions for substance use, medication management, and housing and vocational support provided by a collaborative, multidisciplinary team (Green et al., 2007). A study by Barrowclough et al. demonstrated that integrating care for schizophrenia (including cognitive behavioral therapy and family therapy components) with motivational interviewing for substance use led to overall improvement in patient functioning and an overall decrease in positive symptoms of psychosis, a decrease in symptom exacerbations, and an increase in the percentage of days abstinent from drugs and alcohol (Barrowclough et al., 2001). Contingency management, including providing rewards for sobriety, may also be an effective intervention in this population (Drebing et al., 2005). ACT has also been recommended in treating people with dually diagnosed schizophrenia and substance use disorder. While this intervention has been shown to be more effective in improving quality of life in this population, it may be only marginally more effective in reducing substance abuse when compared to comprehensive service coordination (Drake et al., 1998). Although the evidence base is limited, Twelve-Step programs, like Alcoholics Anonymous and Narcotics Anonymous, may also be effective for the dually diagnosed (Bogenshutz, Geppert, & George, 2010), particularly when the intervention is tailored to those with co-occurring disorders: for example, Double Trouble in Recovery (Vogel et al., 1998).

Nicotine use disorders are exceedingly common among individuals with schizophrenia spectrum disorders, along with the significant burden of medical comorbidities associated with tobacco use. A majority of people with schizophrenia smoke cigarettes, with smoking prevalence often found to exceed 70% in this population (Evins, 2008; Ziedonis & George, 1997; De Leon et al., 2002). Smokers with schizophrenia also tend to be heavily dependent and have lower motivation to quit (George, et al., 2000). Research on smoking cessation in schizophrenia has often focused on pharmacotherapies, with varenicline (Williams et al., 2012), bupropion (Evins et al., 2005), and nicotine replacement (George et al., 2000) showing some efficacy. At the same time, work has also been done in developing smoking cessation groups specially tailored to people with schizophrenia, with some limited success (George et al., 2000; Addington et al., 1998).

Homelessness

According to findings collected and published by SAMHSA in 2011, about 30% of homeless persons have a mental illness, and 50% have co-occurring substance use disorders. SAMHSA also reports that, among homeless veterans, these percentages are even higher, with 45% having mental illness and 70% having substance use disorders (SAMHSA, 2011). In a large study conducted with seriously mentally ill individuals in San Diego, California, the prevalence of homelessness was 15% over a one-year period. Homelessness was most associated with diagnoses of schizophrenia and bipolar disorder and was also correlated with reduced use of outpatient-type services and increased use of inpatient and emergency services (Folsom et al., 2005). In a comprehensive review of schizophrenia and homelessness, which examined studies largely hailing from the United States, Australia, Brazil, and several countries in Europe, the prevalence of schizophrenia in homeless persons was found to be around 11%, with higher rates of schizophrenia found in homeless women and younger adults, as well as in the chronically homeless (Folsom & Jeste, 2002).

Homelessness itself presents specific challenges for the treatment of schizophrenia. Housing First and other supported housing models have been proposed as ways to address housing issues and simultaneously promote or facilitate connection with treatment. Treatment itself might be best addressed in the ACT model, as it has been linked to lower rates of homelessness in at-risk groups, when compared to standard treatment (Dixon et al., 2010).

Incarceration

Patients with a history of mental illness are at high risk for incarceration. According to a U.S. Department of Justice report, in U.S. prisons and jails, more than 450,000 inmates have a recent history of mental illness. This report further finds that, nationwide, nearly a quarter of state prisoners, 21% of jail inmates, and 14% of federal prisoners are mentally ill (James & Glaze, 2006). According to another report, the prevalence of schizophrenia or other psychotic disorders is between 2% and 4% among inmates in state prisons, 0.8% and 2.5% among those incarcerated in federal prison, and 1% among jail inmates (National Commission on Correctional Health Care, 2002). Co-occurring substance use disorders are common among mentally ill inmates, and inmates with a history of substance abuse and serious mental illness are more likely to be charged with violent crimes (McNiel, Binder, & Robinson, 2005; James & Glaze, 2006). The majority of crimes committed by people with serious mental illness, though, may be nonviolent (Fisher et al., 2006; Treatment Advocacy Center, 2009). These nonviolent crimes commonly include offenses like disturbing the peace, shoplifting, and trespassing, as well as certain drug offenses (Fisher et al., 2006). Regardless of crime severity, inmates with severe mental illness and substance use disorders were incarcerated for longer periods than were demographically similar inmates serving sentences for similar crimes (McNiel, Binder, & Robinson, 2005). Recidivism among seriously mentally ill inmates is also particularly high (Baillargeon et al., 2009). Many experts are concerned about the well-being of mentally ill prisoners, citing suicide rates by mentally ill inmates and studies that show that mentally ill prisoners may be at greater risk for victimization by other prisoners (Treatment Advocacy Center, 2009). Mentally ill prisoners also present behavioral challenges that put them and other prisoners and corrections staff at risk (James & Glaze, 2006), and common practices in jails and prisons can lead to worsening symptoms (Treatment Advocacy Center, 2009). The frequent use of solitary confinement for seriously mentally ill inmates is particularly controversial, as it has been linked to psychiatric decompensation and suicide (Metzner & Fellner, 2010).

Some experts have voiced concerns that, in recent years, more and more people with serious mental illness are being incarcerated (Torrey, 2014). Reasons for this are likely to be multifactorial and may include deinstitutionalization, reductions of treatment availability and spending, and, more controversially, barriers to involuntary commitment (The Sentencing Project, 2002). Some advocates, perhaps most vocally the Treatment Advocacy Center (TAC), argue that civil commitments that require patients to engage in outpatient treatment, commonly called *involuntary outpatient commitments, community treatment orders,* or *assisted outpatient treatment* (AOT), can reduce crimes committed by seriously mentally ill individuals, particularly those who have minimal or no insight into their need for treatment. TAC cites the success of New York's Kendra's Law, which incorporates AOT, in reducing incarceration rates among patients on AOT. In addition to reducing rates of incarceration, Kendra's Law has also been cited to have significantly reduced arrests, homelessness, and psychiatric hospitalization (New York State Office of Mental Health, 2012).

Other groups have focused on diverting mentally ill offenders from incarceration, with the President's New Freedom Commission on Mental Health calling for the adoption of adult and juvenile criminal diversion and community re-entry programs to prevent "the unnecessary criminalization and extended incarceration of non-violent adult and juvenile offenders with mental illnesses" (President's New Freedom Commission on Mental Health, 2003). Jail diversion programs are widely thought to decrease the amount of time that mentally ill people, including those with comorbid substance use disorders, spend in jail, without compromising the safety of the community at large. There are over 300 jail diversion programs in the United States, some of which are funded by SAMSHA, others by the Bureau of Justice Assistance. Most programs incorporate either pre- or post-booking diversion strategies.

Pre-booking diversion approaches focus on initial police encounters, before charges are filed. Programs that take this approach include crisis intervention teams (CIT), based on a Memphis program founded in 1988, which call upon specially trained police officers to respond to mental health crisis situations and connect individuals in need with mental health services. When compared to one early study of police interventions in psychiatric emergencies, far fewer police interactions with Memphis CIT led to arrests (Steadman & Naples, 2005). Other pre-booking programs under study feature mental health workers or teams specially trained to work alongside police officers.

Post-booking tactics center on jails or the court system. Appropriate offenders with mental health issues can be diverted before legal charges are filed, during the pretrial period, or during the trial stage itself, if the prosecutor agrees to defer prosecution or sentencing. Diversion can also occur when the offender has violated, or is at risk of violating, probation (GAINS Center for Behavioral Health and Justice Transformation, 2014). The most well-known post-booking diversion tactic is the use of mental health courts, in which select defendants voluntarily plead guilty to criminal charges and agree to a sentence imposed by the court. The terms of this sentence generally involve required mental health treatment and close court follow-up. While defendant eligibility and court jurisdiction vary widely by region, in general, if a mental health court defendant does not comply with the terms of their sentence, they may face legal consequences, including reincarceration and revocation of the original sentence (Steadman et al., 2011). This type of system relies heavily on collaboration between the court and mental health agencies. Some critics worry that mental health courts could abridge defendants' rights, stigmatize them, expand the power of the court system, or divert limited resources from other mental health programs (Clark, 2004). Several studies of mental health courts have shown promising results, though, including a reduction in arrests rate and incarceration days (Steadman et al., 2011).

Release planning for seriously mentally ill inmates from jail or prison is also crucial. Re-entry into a community setting is often a challenge for incarcerated persons, and seriously mentally ill individuals, especially those who have not connected with treatment, may have particular difficulty in obtaining housing and employment (Baillargeon, Hoge, & Penn, 2010). An increasing number of jurisdictions are developing and funding programs to connect seriously mentally ill individuals to treatment post-incarceration, and these initiatives include working to make sure former inmates have health insurance benefits to cover treatment. Forensic assertive community treatment teams and forensic intensive case management services have begun to be deployed, and both are being studied for their effectiveness in addressing the specific needs of this population. The benefits of current programming have not been resoundingly clear, however, and they probably require further development (Morrissey, Meyer, & Cuddeback, 2007).

Involuntary Treatment

In psychiatry, "involuntary treatment" is treating a patient over the patient's objection. It can also involve treatment of a patient who may voice agreement to treatment but who does not have the mental capacity to consent. The most widely utilized type of involuntary psychiatric treatment is involuntary inpatient hospitalization. Indications for inpatient hospitalizations were explored in more depth earlier in this chapter, but generally, hospitalizations are only pursued as a treatment option if outpatient treatment is not sufficient to meet a patient's needs and/or the patient is an imminent danger to themselves or others. If the patient does not agree to hospitalization, or cannot give consent to admission, an emergency psychiatric hospitalization, or "psychiatric hold," can be pursued. This type of hospitalization is often used for psychiatric observation of the patient and usually lasts, at most, for a few days. Involuntary inpatient civil commitments extend for longer periods and are ordered by a judge when recommended by treatment providers and if specific commitment criteria are met. Legal criteria for involuntary inpatient commitment vary widely by state but are generally available throughout the country (Treatment Advocacy Center, 2011).

Involuntary outpatient commitments laws exist in most states. Critics have noted, however, that in several of these states, involuntary outpatient commitments are not actually used (Stettin et al., 2014). The practice of enforcing outpatient commitment laws also varies significantly by state, and even within a state, regional or local interpretations of state law may not be consistent.

New York's Assisted Outpatient Treatment (AOT) protocols may be considered a benchmark in involuntary outpatient commitments. The TAC cites the success of New York's Kendra's Law, a cornerstone of which is AOT, in reducing incarceration rates among patients on AOTs. In addition to reducing rates of incarceration, Kendra's Law has also been cited to have significantly reduced arrests, homelessness, and psychiatric hospitalization (New York State Office of Mental Health, 2012). Like many outpatient commitments, New York's AOT is generally enacted prior to any acts of dangerousness and can thus be considered "preventative" (Swanson & Swartz, 2014). If the patient does not comply with the AOT order, the patient can be transported to a local inpatient mental health facility, where they can be held for observation and treatment for 72 hours before either being released or held on a court-approved involuntary inpatient commitment order.

On a national level, there has been much recent discussion of the potential need to standardize and strengthen outpatient commitment programs, with potentially sweeping mental health legislation, including such provisions' being debated in Washington. Included in this national conversation has been disagreement over both the effectiveness and the ethics of involuntary outpatient treatment. Several studies of outpatient commitments, conducted in North Carolina, Massachusetts, Washington, D.C., Ohio, Tennessee, and Iowa seem to support their efficacy, at least in terms or reducing inpatient hospitalization (Petrila, Ridgely, & Borum, 2003). However, these studies were hampered by methodological limitations, which included a lack of clarity on state outpatient commitment standards, vary-ing levels of treatment intensity, and not including comparison groups. The Cochrane collaborative, for example, found mini-mal evidence to support the efficacy of involuntary outpatient commitments, but they were only able to identify two random-ized control trials for use in their analysis (Kisley, Campbell, & Preston, 2012). These studies had several important limitations, however, and secondary analysis of one of the studies may lend support to the use of outpatient commitments for a select group of individuals with psychotic spectrum disorders. The Oxford Community Treatment Order Evaluation Trial (OCTET) con-ducted in the United Kingdom (Burns, et al., 2013) also cast doubt on the effectiveness of involuntary outpatient commit-ments, as it did not show any difference in rates of hospitaliza-tion between the outpatient involuntary commitment groups and the control condition, nor did it show any differences in secondary outcomes, including length of hospital stay, time to first readmission, or clinical and social functioning. It should be stressed, though, as has been done by other authors (Swanson & Swartz, 2014), that this study compares two conditions that essentially both involve mandated outpatient treatment, with legal means in place through which to hospitalize a patient if the patient did not adhere to the treatment. The question of whether or not involuntary outpatient treatment is more effec-tive than voluntary treatment of the same modality thus appears to remain unanswered.

Finally, and not less importantly, ethical questions about the use of involuntary outpatient treatment abound. Many argue that such programs lead people to avoid engagement in voluntary psychiatric treatment due to fear of losing their personal free-dom. Other arguments against involuntary outpatient commit-ments include the potential diversion of limited resources from voluntary programs to provide involuntary services (Bazelon Center, 2000). Although outpatient commitment laws have so far stood up to legal challenges, there are legal arguments against them that are still worth considering (Allen & Smith, 2001). Generally, the law does not have a compelling interest in pre-venting bad acts, which makes legally mandating treatment for a patient who is not at imminent risk of dangerousness somewhat complicated. The argument of legal competency may also be cited, which holds that, unless individuals are legally determined to not have competence, they have the right to refuse treatment.

Lack of insight into need for treatment does not generally meet the legal definition for "incompetence." The exception to legal competency considerations would be emergencies in which the patient is found to be an imminent danger to themselves or others. These criteria generally meet the threshold for involuntary inpatient psychiatric treatment such that involuntary outpatient treatment becomes a moot point.

Psychiatric Advance Directives

Mental health or psychiatric advance directives have become increasingly popular over the past several years. Just like any advance directive, a mental health advance directive is a document that a patient can prepare when they are competent and have the capacity to make decisions regarding treatment. The document goes into effect when the patient is incapacitated by acute psychiatric illness. Information including crisis symptoms, emergency contacts, and relapse and protective factors can be incorporated into a mental health advance directive, in addition to preferences related to treatment, like medication and hospital choice (National Resource Center for Advance Psychiatric Directives, 2013). Mental health advance directives vary by state in their legal durability, with most states allowing them to be revoked by the authors even when they are incapacitated. Some states do not allow the use of proxy decision makers, who are often named in advance directives, to consent for the patient on specific types mental health treatment (Swanson et al., 2003), including psychiatric hospital admission or electroconvulsive therapy. In addition, existing state laws concerning involuntary treatment can often override the tenets of an advance directive, and physicians in most states can overrule patients' medication preferences when medically appropriate. Patient hospital choice can also be limited by insurance and bed availability.

Guardianship

Rarely, people with severe and chronic mental illness, including some individuals extremely disabled by schizophrenia spectrum disorder, may be determined legally incompetent by a judge. Rendering someone legally incompetent requires that the person in question chronically lack the capacity to make decisions in multiple domains, usually of a personal and/or financial nature, such that another person, or agency, is required to make those decisions for them. The duty of guardians, and the ease with which they can be appointed, is highly dependent on the state in which guardianship is sought. In many states, guardianship is very difficult and expensive to obtain, and the process is always fraught with important ethical considerations. As such, the courts often encourage the pursuit of other measures to help the severely disabled maintain their legal rights of financial and personal decision-making. Such alternatives to guardianship could include retaining a power of attorney, naming a payee to manage social security benefits, or obtaining a financial manager for trusts (DeLosh et al., 2013).

If guardianship is granted by the court, the guardian has to meet a series of qualifications and obligations. In general, guardians are legally responsible with keeping the courts updated about the condition of the person and information as to their finances, medical supports received, and other information pertinent to the guardian's entrusted duties. A guardian may be appointed temporarily or permanently, and endowed with broad or more restricted powers. For example, a "guardian of the estate," who may also be called "guardian of the property" or "conservator," will make all major financial decisions for the incapacitated person, including but not limited to selling or obtaining property, paying bills, and managing trusts. A "guardian of the person," rarely also called a "conservator," can generally make medical decisions for the incapacitated person, but they may not be allowed to commit someone to a psychiatric hospital if the patient does not meet grounds for involuntary commitment. A "full" or "unlimited guardian" will generally be charged with making both personal and financial decisions for the incapacitated persons. Note that incapacitated persons are also sometimes called "wards," "conservatees," or "protected persons."

Conclusion

Patient-centered treatment of schizophrenia and related psychotic disorders includes thoughtful consideration of available psychosocial treatments, not just for the management of psychotic symptoms, but to help facilitate patient recovery. Existing systems of care, spanning inpatient and outpatient modalities, must be navigated carefully to promote effective treatment. Specific psychosocial approaches called upon by patients and their providers may be associated with housing, incorporate case management, and involve the use of specific psychotherapies. Common challenges in treatment should be recognized by providers, and evidence-based, psychosocial approaches to treatment barriers should be explored.

Self-Learning Questions

1. The goals of "recovery," in mental health:
    a. Usually include discontinuation of treatment
    b. Often focus on positive coping, building resilience, and empowerment
    c. Are highly individualized, strength-based, and embrace social connectedness
    d. b and c
    e. All of the above

2. Assertive Community Treatment (ACT):
    a. Increases the duration of patients' hospital stays
    b. Decreases housing stability
    c. Incorporates large caseloads of patients for ACT physicians
    d. Serves patients in an office-based setting
    e. May involve certified peer specialists

3. In terms of housing options, patients with schizophrenia:
    a. Can never live independently
    b. Should not reside with family members
    c. May live in transitional housing with decreasing levels of formal support as they advance in their recovery
    d. Should not reside in supported housing without having first been involved in treatment

4. Cognitive remediation:
    a. Involves repeated or strategic practice at cognitive exercises
    b. Only addresses deficits in non-social cognition
    c. Never involves small groups
    d. Generally relies on pencil and paper testing of free word associations

Key Learning Points

- Psychiatric services for patients with psychotic disorders are provided in inpatient and outpatient settings. Most patients with psychosis can be treated successfully as outpatients during most phases of their illness. Treatment intensity and scope must be tailored to individual patient need, which often changes over time.
- Psychosocial interventions encompassing case management and addressing housing needs can be helpful to ensure community integration.
- Psychotherapy is fundamental in the treatment of patients with psychotic disorders. Evidence-based psychotherapies include supportive therapy, family and patient psychoeducation, social skills training, supported employment, cognitive behavioral therapy for psychosis, and cognitive remediation.

References

Addington, J., El-Guebaly, N., Campbell, W., Hodgins, D. C., & Addington, D. (1998). Smoking cessation treatment for patients with schizophrenia. *The American Journal of Psychiatry, 155*(7), 974–975.

Allen, M. H., Forster, P., Zealberg, J., & Currier, G. (2002). *Report and Recommendations Regarding American Psychiatric Association Task Force on Emergency Psychiatry: Psychiatric Emergency and Crisis Services, A Review and Model Program Descriptions.* Washington, DC: American Psychiatric Association.

Allen, M., & Smith, V. F. (2001). Opening Pandora's box: The practical and legal dangers of involuntary outpatient commitment. *Psychiatric Services, 52*(3), 342–346.

Anderson, C. M., Hogarty, G. E., & Reiss, D. J. (1980). Family treatment of adult schizophrenic patients: A psycho-educational approach. *Schizophrenia Bulletin, 6*(3), 490–505.

Anderson, C. M., Reiss, D. J., & Hogarty, G. E. (1986). *Schizophrenia and the Family.* New York: Guilford.

Anthony, W. A. (1993). Recovery from mental illness: The guiding vision of the mental health service system in the 1990s. *Psychosocial Rehabilitation Journal, 24*(2), 11–23.

Anthony, W., & Farkas, M. (2009). *Primer on the Psychiatric Rehabilitation Process.* Boston, MA: Boston University Center of Psychiatric Rehabilitation.

Baillargeon, J., Binswanger, I. A., Penn, J. V., Williams, B. A., & Murray, O. J. (2009). Psychiatric disorders and repeat incarcerations: The revolving prison door. *American Journal of Psychiatry, 166*(1), 103–109.

Baillargeon, J., Hoge, S. K., & Penn, J. V. (2010). Addressing the challenge of community reentry among released inmates with serious mental illness. *American Journal of Community Psychology, 46*(3–4), 361–375.

Barrowclough, C., Haddock, G., Tarrier, N., Lewis, S. W., Moring, J., O'Brien, R., et al. (2001). Randomized controlled trial of motivational interviewing, cognitive behavioral therapy, and family intervention for patients with comorbid schizophrenia and substance use disorders. *American Journal of Psychiatry, 158*(10), 1706–1713.

Bazelon Center. (2000). *Position Statement on Involuntary Commitment.* Washington, DC: Judge David L. Bazelon Center for Mental Health Law.

Beck, A. T. (1964). Thinking and depression: II. Theory and therapy. *Archives of General Psychiatry, 10*(6), 561–571.

Becker, D., Whitley, R., Bailey, E., & Drake, R. (2007). Long-term employment trajectories among participants with severe mental illness in supported employment. *Psychiatric Services, 58*(7), 922–928.

Bellack, A. S. (2006). Scientific and consumer models of recovery in schizophrenia: Concordance, contrasts, and implications. *Schizophrenia Bulletin, 32*(3), 432–442.

Bellack, A. S., Mueser, K. T., Gingerich, S., & Agresta, J. (2004). *Social Skills Training for Schizophrenia: A Step-by-Step Guide.* New York: Guilford.

Bogenshutz, M. P., Geppert, C., & George, J. (2010). The role of Twelve-Step approaches in dual diagnosis treatment and recovery. *The American Journal on Addictions, 15*(1), 50–60.

Bond, G. R. (1998). Principles of the Individual Placement and Support model: Empirical support. *Psychiatric Rehabilitation Journal, 22*(1), 11–23.

Bond, G., Drake, R., & Becker, D. R. B. (2008). An update on randomized controlled trials of evidence-based supported employment. *Psychiatric Rehabilitation Journal, 31*(4), 280–290.

Buchanan, R. W., Javitt, D. C., Marder, S. R., Schooler, N. R., Gold, J. M., McMahon, R. P., et al. (2007). The Cognitive and Negative Symptoms in Schizophrenia Trial (CONSIST): The efficacy of glutamatergic agents for negative symptoms and cognitive impairments. *American Journal of Psychiatry*, 164(10), 1593–1602.

Buckley, L. A., Pettit, T., & Adams, C. E. (2007). Supportive therapy for schizophrenia. *The Cochrane Database of Systematic Reviews*, 3, CD004716.

Burns, A. M., Erickson, D. H., & Brenner, C. A. (2014). Cognitive-behavioral therapy for medication-resistant psychosis: A meta-analytic review. *Psychiatric Services*, 65(7), 874–880.

Burns, T., Catty, J., Becker, T., Drake, R. E., Fioritti, A., Knapp, M., et al. (2007). The effectiveness of supported employment for people with severe mental illness: A randomised controlled trial. *Lancet*, 370(9593), 1146–1152.

Burns, T., Rugkasa, J., Molodynski, A., Dawson, J., Yeeles, K., Vazquez-Montes, M., et al. (2013). Community treatment orders for patients with psychosis (OCTET): A randomised controlled trial. *Lancet*, 381(9878), 1627–1633.

Butler, A. C., Chapman, J. E., Forman, E. M., & Beck, A. T. (2006). The empirical status of cognitive-behavioral therapy: A review of meta-analyses. *Clinical Psychology Review*, 26(1), 17–31.

Butzlaff, R. L., & Hooley, J. M. (1998). Expressed emotion and psychiatric relapse: A meta-analysis. *Archives of General Psychiatry*, 55(6), 547–552.

Campbell, K., Bond, G. R., & Drake, R. E. (2011). Who benefits from supported employment: A meta-analytic study. *Schizophrenia Bulletin*, 37(2), 370–380.

Clark, J. (2004). *Non-Speciality First Appearance Court Models for Diverting Persons with Mental Illness: Alternatives to Mental Health Courts*. Delmar, NY: Technical Assistance and Policy Analysis Center for Jail Diversion.

Cohen, M. R., Farkas, M. D., & Gange, C. (2002). *Psychiatric Rehabilitation*. Boston, MA: Center for Psychiatric Rehabilitation, Sargent College of Health and Rehabilitation Sciences, Boston University.

Cramer, S. C., & Riley, J. D. (2008). Neuroplasticity and brain repair after stroke. *Current Opinion in Neurology*, 21(1), 76–82.

De Leon, J., McCann, T., McGory, A., & Diaz, F. (2002). Schizophrenia and tobacco smoking: A replication study in another US psychiatric hospital. *Schizophrenia Research*, 56(1), 55–65.

DeLosh, P., Boyko, C., Cano, E., Corson, T., Dibble, T., Holandez, P., et al. (2013–2014). Adult guardianship guide: A guide to plan, develop, and sustain a comprehensive court guardianship and conservatorship program. Williamsburg, VA: National Association for Court Management.

Diehl, S., Douglas, D., Gay, K., & Hart, J. (2014). *Road to Recovery: Employment and Mental Illness*. Arlington, VA: National Alliance on Mental Illness.

Dieterich, M., Irving, C., Park, B., & Marshall, M. (2010). Intensive case management for severe mental illness (review). *Cochrane Database of Systematic Reviews*, 2010(10), 1–244.

Dixon, L. (1999). Dual diagnosis of substance abuse in schizophrenia: Prevalence and impact on outcomes. *Schizophrenia Research*, 35, S93–S100.

Dixon, L. B., Dickerson, F., Bellack, A. S., Bennett, M., Dickinson, D., Goldberg, R. W., et al. (2010). The 2009 schizophrenia PORT psychosocial treatment recommendations and summary statements. *Schizophrenia Bulletin*, 36(1), 48–70.

Dixon, L., Stewart, B., Burland, J., Delahanty, J., Lucksted, A., & Hoffman, M. (2001). Pilot study of the effectiveness of the family-to-family education program. *Psychiatric Services*, 52(7), 965–967.

Drake, R. E., McHugo, G. J., Clark, R. E., Teague, G. B., Xie, H., Miles, K., et al. (1998). Assertive community treatment for patients with co-occurring severe mental illness and substance use disorder: A clinical trial. *American Journal of Orthopsychiatry*, 68(2), 201–215.

Drebing, C., Van Ormer, E. A., Krebs, C., Rosenheck, R., Rounsaville, B., Herz, L., et al. (2005). The impact of enhanced incentives on vocational rehabilitation outcomes for dually diagnosed veterans. *Journal of Applied Behavioral Analysis*, 38(3), 359–372.

Druss, B. G., Rohrbaugh, R. M., Levinson, C. M., & Rosenheck, R. A. (2001). Integrated medical care for patients with serious psychiatric illness: A randomized trial. *Archives of General Psychiatry*, 58(9), 861–868.

Eack, S. M. (2012). Cognitive remediation: A new generation of psychosocial interventions for people with schizophrenia. *Social Work*, 57(3), 235–246.

Eack, S. M., Greenwald, D. P., Hogarty, S. S., Cooley, S. J., DiBarry, A. L., Montrose, D. M., et al. (2009). Cognitive enhancement therapy for early-course schizophrenia: Effects of a two-year randomized controlled trial. *Psychiatric Services*, 60(11), 1468–1476.

Eack, S. M., Hogarty, G. E., Cho, R. Y., Prasad, K. M. R., Greenwald, D. P., Hogarty, S. S., et al. (2010). Neuroprotective effects of cognitive enhancement therapy against gray matter loss in early schizophrenia: Results from a two-year randomized controlled trial. *Archives of General Psychiatry*, 67(7), 674–682.

Evins, A. E. (2008, March 1). Nicotine dependence in schizophrenia: Prevalence, mechanisms, and implications for treatment. *Psychiatric Times*. Retrieved from http://www.psychiatrictimes.com/schizophrenia/nicotine-dependence-schizophrenia-prevalence-mechanisms-and-implications-treatment/page/0/2.

Evins, A. E., Cather, C., Deckersbach, T., Freudenreich, O., Culhane, M., Olm-Shipman, C. M., et al. (2005). A double-blind placebo-controlled trial of bupropion sustained-release for smoking cessation in schizophrenia. *Journal of Clinical Psychopharmacology*, 25(3), 218–225.

Fisher, W. H., Roy-Bujnowski, K. M., Grudzinskas, A. J., Clayfield, J. C., Banks, S. M., & Wolff, N. (2006). Patterns and prevalence of arrest in a statewide cohort of mental health care consumers. *Psychiatric Services*, 57(11), 1623–1628.

Fleishman, M. (2004). Economic grand rounds: The problem: How many patients live in residential care facilities? *Psychiatric Services*, 55(6), 620–622.

Folsom, D. P., Hawthorne, W., Lindamer, L., Gilmer, T., Bailey, A., Golshan, S., et al. (2005). Prevalence and risk factors for homelessness and utilization of mental health services among 10,340 patients with serious mental illness in a large public mental health system. *The American Journal of Psychiatry*, 162(2), 370–376.

Folsom, D., & Jeste, D. (2002). Schizophrenia in homeless persons: A systematic review of the literature. *Acta Psychiatrica Scandinavica*, 105(6), 404–413.

Fowler, I. L., Carr, V. J., Carter, N. T., & Lewin, T. J. (1998). Patterns of current and lifetime substance use in schizophrenia. *Schizophrenia Bulletin*, 24(3), 443–455.

GAINS Center for Behavioral Health and Justice Transformation. (2014). *Types of Jail Diversion*. Rockville, MD: Substance Abuse and Mental Health Services Administration. Retrieved from http://gainscenter.samhsa.gov/topical_resources/jail.asp.

George, T. P., Ziedonis, D. M., Feingold, A., Pepper, T., Satterburg, C. A., Winkel, J., et al. (2000). Nicotine transdermal patch and atypical antipsychotic medications for smoking cessation in schizophrenia. *American Journal of Psychiatry*, 157(11), 1835–1842.

Green, A. I., Drake, R. E., Brunette, M. F., & Noordsy, D. L. (2007). Treatment in psychiatry: Schizophrenia and co-occurring substance use disorder. *American Journal of Psychiatry*, 164(3), 402–408.

Heinrichs, R. W., & Zakzanis, K. K. (1998). Neurocognitive deficit in schizophrenia: A quantitative review of the evidence. *Neuropsychology*, 12(3), 426–445.

Hogan, M. F. (2003). New Freedom Commission Report: The President's New Freedom Commission: Recommendations to transform mental health care in America. *Psychiatric Services, 54*(11), 1467–1474.

Hogarty, G. E. (2002). *Personal Therapy for Schizophrenia and Related Disorders: A Guide to Individualized Treatment.* New York: Guilford.

Hogarty, G. E., & Greenwald, D. P. (2006). *Cognitive Enhancement Therapy: The Training Manual.* Pittsburgh, PA: University of Pittsburgh Medical Center. Retrieved from www.CognitiveEnhancementTherapy.com.

Hogarty, G. E., Anderson, C. M., Reiss, D. J., Kornblith, S. J., Greenwald, D. P., Javna, C. D., et al., & the Environmental/Personal Indicators in the Course of Schizophrenia (EPICS) Research Group. (1986). Family psychoeducation, social skills training, and maintenance chemotherapy in the aftercare treatment of schizophrenia: I. One-year effects of a controlled study on relapse and expressed emotion. *Archives of General Psychiatry, 43*(7), 633–642.

Hogarty, G. E., Anderson, C. M., Reiss, D. J., Kornblith, S. J., Greenwald, D. P., Ulrich, R. F., et al., & the Environmental/Personal Indicators in the Course of Schizophrenia (EPICS) Research Group. (1991). Family psychoeducation, social skills training, and maintenance chemotherapy in the aftercare treatment of schizophrenia: II. Two-year effects of a controlled study on relapse and adjustment. *Archives of General Psychiatry, 48*(4), 340–347.

Hogarty, G. E., Flesher, S., Ulrich, R., Carter, M., Greenwald, D., Pogue-Geile, M., et al. (2004). Cognitive enhancement therapy for schizophrenia. Effects of a 2-year randomized trial on cognition and behavior. *Archives of General Psychiatry, 61*(9), 866–876.

Hogarty, G. E., Goldberg, S. C., Schooler, N. R., & the Collaborative Study Group. (1974b). Drug and sociotherapy in the aftercare of schizophrenic patients: III. Adjustment of nonrelapsed patients. *Archives of General Psychiatry, 31*(5), 609–618.

Hogarty, G. E., Goldberg, S. C., Schooler, N. R., Ulrich, R. F., & the Collaborative Study Group. (1974a). Drug and sociotherapy in the aftercare of schizophrenic patients. II. Two-year relapse rates. *Archives of General Psychiatry, 31*(5), 603–608.

Hogarty, G. E., Greenwald, D., Ulrich, R. F., Kornblith, S. J., Dibarry, A. L., Cooley, S., et al. (1997b). Three-year trials of personal therapy among schizophrenic patients living with or independent of family: II. Effects on adjustment of patients. *American Journal of Psychiatry, 154*(11), 1514–1524.

Hogarty, G. E., Kornblith, S. J., Greenwald, D., Dibarry, A. L., Cooley, S., Ulrich, R. F., et al. (1997a). Three-year trials of personal therapy among schizophrenic patients living with or independent of family: I. Description of study and effects of relapse rates. *American Journal of Psychiatry, 154*(11), 1504–1513.

James, D. J., & Glaze, L. E. (2006). *Bureau of Justice Statistics Special Report: Mental Health Problems of Prison and Jail Inmates.* Washington, DC: U.S. Department of Justice, Office of Justice Programs.

Jauhar, S., McKenna, P. J., Radua, J., Fung, E., Salvador, R., & Laws, K. R. (2014). Cognitive-behavioural therapy for the symptoms of schizophrenia: Systematic review and meta-analysis with examination of potential bias. *British Journal of Psychiatry, 204*(1), 20–29.

Keefe, R. S. E., Bilder, R. M., Davis, S. M., Harvey, P. D., Palmer, B. W., Gold, J. M., et al. (2007). Neurocognitive effects of antipsychotic medications in patients with chronic schizophrenia in the CATIE trial. *Archives of General Psychiatry, 64*(6), 633–647.

Kingdon, D. G., & Turkington, D. (1994). *Cognitive-Behavioral Therapy of Schizophrenia.* New York: Guilford.

Kisley, S., Campbell, L., & Preston, N. (2012). Compulsory community and involuntary outpatient treatment for people with severe mental disorders (review). *The Cochrane Database of Systematic Reviews*, 2012 (10), 1–44.

Kurtz, M. M., & Mueser, K. T. (2008). A meta-analysis of controlled research on social skills training for schizophrenia. *Journal of Consulting and Clinical Psychology*, 76(3), 491–504.

Kurtz, M. M., & Richardson, C. L. (2012). Social cognitive training for schizophrenia: A meta-analytic investigation of controlled research. *Schizophrenia Bulletin*, 38(5), 1092–1104.

Lehman, A., Lieberman, J., Dixon, L., McGlashan, T., Miller, A., Perkins, D., et al. (2004). Practice guidelines for the treatment of patients with schizophrenia, 2nd ed. *The American Journal of Psychiatry*, 161(2 Suppl), 1–56.

Lincoln, T. M., Wilhelm, K., & Nestoriuc, Y. (2007). Effectiveness of psychoeducation for relapse, symptoms, knowledge, adherence and functioning in psychotic disorders: A meta-analysis. *Schizophrenia Research*, 96(1), 232–245.

Marder, S. R., Wirshing, W. C., Mintz, J., McKenzie, J., Johnston, K., Eckman, T. A., et al. (1996). Two-year outcome of social skills training and group psychotherapy for outpatients with schizophrenia. *American Journal of Psychiatry*, 153(12), 1585–1592.

Marshall, M., Crowther, R., Almaraz-Serrano, A., Sledge, W., Kluiter, H., Robert, C., et al. (2003). Day hospital versus admission for acute psychiatric disorders. *The Cochrane Database of Systematic Reviews*, 2011(12), 1–41.

Marwaha, S., & Johnson, S. (2004). Schizophrenia and employment: A review. *Social Psychiatry and Psychiatric Epidemiology*, 39(5), 337–349.

Marx, G., & Jackson, D. (2012, July 4). Illinois struggles to move mentally ill adults out of nursing homes. *Chicago Tribune*. Retrieved from http://articles.chicago-tribune.com/2012-07-04/health/ct-met-nursing-home-report-20120704_1_nursing-homes-state-officials-consent-decree

McFarlane, W. R., Lukens, E., Link, B., Dushay, R., Deakins, S. A., Newmark, M., et al. (1995). Multiple-family groups and psychoeducation in the treatment of schizophrenia. *Archives of General Psychiatry*, 52(8), 679–687.

McGurk, S. R., Twamley, E. W., Sitzer, D. I., McHugo, G. J., & Mueser, K. T. (2007). A meta-analysis of cognitive remediation in schizophrenia. *American Journal of Psychiatry*, 164(12), 1791–1802.

McNiel, D. E., Binder, R., & Robinson, J. C. (2005). Incarceration associated with homelessness, mental disorder, and co-occurring substance abuse. *Psychiatric Services*, 56(7), 840–846.

Messer, S. B., & Wampold, B. E. (2002). Let's face facts: Common factors are more potent than specific therapy ingredients. *Clinical Psychology Science and Practice*, 9(1), 21–25.

Metzner, J., & Fellner, J. (2010). Solitary confinement and mental illness in U.S. prisons: A challenge for medical ethics. *Journal of the American Academy of Psychiatry and the Law*, 38(1), 104–108.

Morrison, A. P., French, P., Walford, L., Lewis, S. W., Kilcommons, A., Green, J., et al. (2004). Cognitive therapy for the prevention of psychosis in people at ultra-high risk: Randomised controlled trial. *British Journal of Psychiatry*, 185(4), 291–297.

Morrissey, J., Meyer, P., & Cuddeback, G. (2007). Extending assertive community treatment to criminal justice settings: Origins, current evidence, and future directions. *Community Mental Health Journal*, 38(1), 527–544.

Mueser, K. T., & Tarrier, N. (1998). *Handbook of Social Functioning in Schizophrenia*. Boston, MA: Allyn and Bacon.

290 Schizophrenia and Related Disorders

Mueser, K. T., Bellack, A. S., Douglas, M. S., & Morrison, R. L. (1991). Prevalence and stability of social skill deficits in schizophrenia. *Schizophrenia Research, 5*(2), 167–176.

Mueser, K. T., Corrigan, P. W., Hilton, D. W., Tanzman, B., Schaub, A., Gingerich, S., et al. (2002). Illness management and recovery: A review of the research. *Psychiatric Services, 53*(10), 1272–1284.

Mueser, K. T., Deavers, F., Penn, D. L., & Cassisi, J. E. (2013). Psychosocial treatments for schizophrenia. *Annual Review of Clinical Psychology, 9*(1), 465–497.

Mueser, K. T., Sengupta, A., Schooler, N. R., Bellack, A. S., Xie, H., Glick, I. D., et al. (2001). Family treatment and medication dosage reduction in schizophrenia: Effects on patient social functioning, family attitudes, and burden. *Journal of Consulting and Clinical Psychology, 69*(1), 3–12.

Murphy, S., Irving, C.B., Adams, C.E., & Driver, R. (2012). Crisis intervention for people with severe mental illnesses. *Schizophrenia Bulletin, 38*(4), 676–677.

National Alliance on Mental Illness. (2007). Assertive Community Treatment: Investment yields outcomes. Retrieved from http://www.nami.org/Template.cfm?Section=act_ta_center&template=/ContentManagement/ContentDisplay.cfm&ContentID=52382. Arlington, VA: National Alliance for Mental Illness. (April 25, 2014)

National Commission on Correctional Health Care. (2002). *The Health Status of Soon-to-Be-Released Inmates, A Report to Congress,* Vol. 1. Washington, DC: National Commission on Correctional Health Care.

National Resource Center on Advance Psychiatric Directives. (2013). *What Information Goes into Psychiatric Advance Directives?* [Motion picture]. NC: National Resource Center on Advance Psychiatric Directives.

New York State Office of Mental Health. (2012). *Kendra's Law: Final Report on the Status of Assisted Outpatient Treatment.* Albany, NY: New York State Office of Mental Health.

New York Times. (2002, April 30). The adult home scandal. *New York Times.* Retrieved from http://www.nytimes.com/2002/04/30/opinion/the-adult-home-scandal.html

Penn, D. L., Corrigan, P. W., Bentall, R. P., Racenstein, J., & Newman, L. (1997). Social cognition in schizophrenia. *Psychological Bulletin, 121*(1), 114–132.

Penn, D. L., Meyer, P. S., Evans, E., Wirth, R. J., Cai, K., & Burchinal, M. (2009). A randomized controlled trial of group cognitive-behavioral therapy vs. enhanced supportive therapy for auditory hallucinations. *Schizophrenia Research, 109*(1), 52–59.

Penn, D. L., Mueser, K. T., Tarrier, N., Gloege, A., Cather, C., Serrano, D., et al. (2004). Supportive therapy for schizophrenia. *Schizophrenia Bulletin, 30*(1), 101–112.

Petrila, J., Ridgely, M. S., & Borum, R. (2003). Debating outpatient commitment: Controversy, trends, and empirical data. *Crime and Delinquency, 49*(1), 157–172.

Pitschel-Walz, G., Leucht, S., Bäuml, J., Kissling, W., & Engel, R. R. (2001). The effect of family interventions on relapse and rehospitalization in schizophrenia—a meta-analysis. *Schizophrenia Bulletin, 27*(1), 73–92.

President's New Freedom Commission on Mental Health. (2003). *Achieving the Promise: Transforming Mental Health Care in America.* Rockville, MD: President's New Freedom Commission on Mental Health.

Rogers, E., Kash-MacDonald, M., & Olschewski, A. (2009). *Systematic Review of Supported Housing Literature, 1993–2008.* Boston, MA: Boston University, Sargent College, Center for Psychiatric Rehabilitation.

Rotondi, A., Anderson, C., Haas, G., Eack, S., Spring, M., Ganguli, R., et al. (2010). Web-based psychoeducational intervention for persons with schizophrenia and their supporters: One-year outcomes. *Psychiatric Services*, 61(11), 1099–1105.

SAMHSA-HRSA. (2012). *Behavioral Health Homes for People with Mental Health and Substance Use Conditions—Core Clinical Features*. Washington, DC: SAMHSA-HRSA Center for Integrated Health Solutions.

Sentencing Project, The. (2002). *Mentally Ill Offenders in the Criminal Justice System: An Analysis and Prescription*. Washington, DC: The Sentencing Project.

Soyka, M., Albus, M., Kathmann, N., Finelli, A., Holzback, R., Immler, B., et al. (1992). Prevalence of alcohol and drug abuse in schizophrenic inpatients. *European Archive of Psychiatry and Clinical Neuroscience*, 242(6), 362–372.

Steadman, H. J., & Naples, M. (2005). Assessing the effectiveness of jail diversion programs for persons with serious mental illness and co-occurring substance use disorders. *Behavioral Sciences and the Law*, 23(2), 163–170.

Steadman, H. J., Mulvey, E. P., Monahan, J., Robbins, P. C., Appelbaum, P. S., Grisso, T., et al. (1998). Violence by people discharged from acute psychiatric inpatient facilities and by others in the same neighborhoods. *Archives of General Psychiatry*, 55(5), 393–401.

Steadman, H. J., Redlich, A., Callahan, L., Robbins, P. C., & Vesselinov, R. (2011). Effect of mental health courts on arrests and jail days: A multisite study. *Archives of General Psychiatry*, 68(2), 162–172.

Stein, L., & Test, M. A. (1980). Alternative to mental hospital treatment: I. Conceptual model, treatment program, and clinical evaluation. *Archives of General Psychiatry*, 37(4), 392–397.

Stettin, B., Geller, J., Ragosta, K., Cohen, K., & Ghowrwal, J. (2014). *Mental Health Commitment Laws: A Survey of the States*. Arlington, VA: Treatment Advocacy Center.

Subramaniam, K., Luks, T. L., Fisher, M., Simpson, G. V., Nagarajan, S., & Vinogradov, S. (2012). Computerized cognitive training restores neural activity within the reality monitoring network in schizophrenia. *Neuron*, 73(4), 842–853.

Substance Abuse and Mental Health Services Administration. (2005). *National Consensus on Mental Health Recovery and Systems Transformation*. Rockville, MD: Department of Health and Human Services.

Substance Abuse and Mental Health Services Administration. (2011). *Current Statistics on the Prevalence and Characteristics of People Experiencing Homelessness in the United States*. Washington, DC: Substance Abuse and Mental Health Services Administration.

Swanson, J., & Swartz, M. (2014). Why the evidence for outpatient commitment is good enough. *Psychiatric Services*, 65(6), 808–811.

Swanson, J., Swartz, M., Hannon, M., & Elbogen, E. (2003). Psychiatric advance directives: A survey of persons with schizophrenia, family members, and treatment providers. *International Journal of Forensic Mental Health*, 2(1), 73–86.

Tarrier, N., Kinney, C., McCarthy, E., Humphreys, L., Wittkowski, A., & Morris, J. (2000). Two-year follow-up of cognitive-behavioral therapy and supportive counseling in the treatment of persistent symptoms in chronic schizophrenia. *Journal of Consulting and Clinical Psychology*, 68(5), 917–922.

Torrey, E. F. (2014). *Bedlam Revisited: Jails, Police, and Mental Health Courts as the New Psychiatric Care*. New York: American Psychiatric Association.

Treatment Advocacy Center. (2009). *Jails and Prisons*. Arlington, VA: Treatment Advocacy Center.

Treatment Advocacy Center. (2011). *State Standards Charts for Assisted Treatment: Civil Commitment Criteria and Initiation Procedures by State*. Arlington, VA: Treatment Advocacy Center (www.TreatmentAdvocacyCenter.org).

Tsemberis, S., & Eisenberg, R. (2000). Pathways to housing: Supported housing for street-dwelling homeless individuals with psychiatric disabilities. *Psychiatric Services, 51*(4), 487–493.

Twamley, E. W., Jeste, D. V., & Lehman, A. F. (2003). Vocational rehabilitation in schizophrenia and other psychotic disorders: A literature review and meta-analysis of randomized controlled trials. *Journal of Nervous and Mental Disease, 191*(8), 515–523.

Vogel, H. S., Knight, E., Laudet, A., & Magura, S. (1998). Double trouble in recovery: Self-help for people with dual diagnoses. *Psychiatry Rehabilitation Journal, 21*(4), 356–364.

Wallace, C. J., & Liberman, R. P. (1985). Social skills training for patients with schizophrenia: A controlled clinical trial. *Psychiatry Research, 15*(3), 239–247.

Wallace, C. J., Nelson, C. J., Liberman, R. P., Aitchison, R. A., Lukoff, D., Elder, J. P., et al. (1980). A review and critique of social skills training with schizophrenic patients. *Schizophrenia Bulletin, 6*(1), 42–63.

Williams, J., Anthenelli, R., Morris, C., Treadow, J., Thompson, J., Yunis, C., et al. (2012). A randomized, double-blind, placebo-controlled study evaluating the safety and efficacy of varenicline for smoking cessation in patients with schizophrenia or schizoaffective disorder. *The Journal of Clinical Psychiatry, 73*(5), 654–660.

Wykes, T., Brammer, M., Mellers, J., Bray, P., Reeder, C., Williams, C., et al. (2002). Effects on the brain of a psychological treatment: Cognitive remediation therapy: Functional magnetic resonance imaging in schizophrenia. *British Journal of Psychiatry, 181*(2), 144–152.

Wykes, T., Huddy, V., Cellard, C., McGurk, S. R., & Czobor, P. (2011). A meta-analysis of cognitive remediation for schizophrenia: Methodology and effect sizes. *American Journal of Psychiatry, 168*(5), 472–485.

Xiong, W., Phillips, M. R., Hu, X., Wang, R., Dai, Q., Kleinman, J., et al. (1994). Family-based intervention for schizophrenic patients in China. A randomised controlled trial. *British Journal of Psychiatry, 165*(2), 239–247.

Ziedonis, D. M., & George, T. P. (1997). Schizophrenia and nicotine use: Report of a pilot smoking cessation program and review of neurobiological and clinical issues. *Schizophrenia Bulletin, 23*(2), 247–254.

Answers

Chapter 1

1 d

2 a

3 e

4 d

5 d

6 e

Chapter 2

1 c

2 c

3 d

4 c

Chapter 3

1 e

2 e

3 c

4 d

Chapter 4

1 e

2 e

3 b

4 d

Chapter 5

1 a

2 c

3 a

4 b

Chapter 6

1 d

2 a

3 a

4 d

5 b

6 a

7 e

Chapter 7

1 d

2 e

3 c

4 a

Index